A unique
SEVENTY YEAR
EXPERIMENT
in PERSONAL HEALTH and
CONSISTENT PHYSICAL
TRAINING leading to
INTERNATIONAL
SPORTING ATTAINMENT

BY Mike Harris

Typeset in ITC Galliard Pro

Editing, design, typesetting and publishing by UK Book Publishing

www.ukbookpublishing.com

ISBN: 978-1-914195-96-9

Oh no, not another health guide? No, you're right, at least not in the conventional sense, this is just me and I'm probably a lot like you, offering a friendly 'crack' on a level designed to be understandable. What follows is based on an entire life of amateur sporting and recreational activity, which has nothing to do with handed down *'research has indicated'* or *'studies have shown'* or *'scientific analysis and experimentation has proven'* or *'recent data shows'*. Furthermore, the book is not about making money; honestly it's true, I don't expect to make a single bronze penny. I've written it firstly because I can, and secondly it all interests me, the subject is one of my engaging hobbies! There are no 'answers' by the way, now that's an author's suicide note, but again it's true! We discuss a variety of subjects – and you choose based on what makes sense and what doesn't!

To all the Professors of', the Physiologists, Dietitians and Sports Nutritionists, Doctors of' and even the Personal Trainers to the 'Stars'!

'Go on; look at my 70 year CV; then tell me I got it all wrong'!!!!

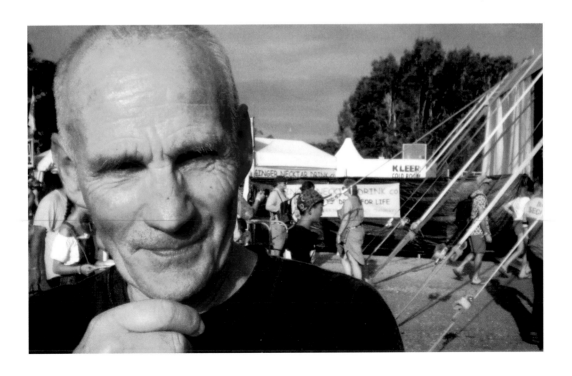

I'm hoping this book will be as unpredictable as my past 70 years have been, and unpredictability may arouse interest and maybe even be the spur that has the reader turning to the next page, if only out of curiosity. The page that follows ('Who are you?') has little to do with the subject of health; however, as I begin writing it's a frustrating example of life in 2021 UK.

Who are you?

Have you ever seen Clint Eastwood in the 'High Plains Drifter'? At the very end of the film, having shot some bad guys, he finally shoots the one remaining bad-ass, it's fatal; I mean Clint doesn't miss now, does he; presumably that's why he's paid so much! Anyhow, as the dying bad guy's life ebbs away in the blood soaked sand and he's on his way to meet his maker, he takes one last look at his nemesis before uttering for the last time a tormented 'who are you?' before he dies!

And here am I, in March 2021, repeatedly saying the same three-word phrase and I have to admit that almost daily I repetitively pose the same question ('who are you') in the same tormented voice as the bandit; mine though is aimed at all those anonymous, well-hidden, seemingly non-existent people who tell me (and you) what you and I can say and more importantly what we can't say. Terms I've used all my *three score years and ten* lifespan are no longer permissible and with the nod of someone's 'educated' and no doubt 'expensive' head, increasingly my very liberal views are henceforth eradicated from any informal discussion, and worse still they disappear without as much as a 'what's your view on that then, Mike?'. So, I'll ask again, 'Who the hell are you?' and with what authority do you have that gives you the absolute right (I mean did I vote you in – to represent me?) to tell me, a good and loyal servant, tax paying, and trouble free citizen of the once free-est and bravest nation in the world, just what I'm permitted to say in life's engaging discussions? I mean 'chest feeding instead of breast feeding' and the British army banning the term 'lads' (wonder how that'll go down in the Stadium of Light?), amongst many others, if I or millions of my country folk had come out with those 'directives', we'd be sectioned. I'll say it again 'who are you?'. Wonder if Clint wants another job?

Let me just give a casual warning, before you consider reading further into this book, there may be personal views which in the wrong hands will see me off to jail, individual perception of detail can be misread resulting in a wrong or unintended interpretation. Regardless, I'd welcome visitors, by appointment please! Richard Littlejohn for Prime Minister – are you with me?

THIS BOOK COULD UNDENIABLY BE CLASSED AS A ONE WAY 'DISCUSSION' REVOLVING AROUND THE SUBJECTS OF HEALTH AND FITNESS. MY VIEWS, OF COURSE, DON'T MAKE ME RIGHT, OR WRONG FOR THAT MATTER, BUT I FEEL THERE IS MUCH EVIDENCE TO AT LEAST SUGGEST I GOT A LOT RIGHT IN MY SEVENTY SWEAT-SOAKED YEARS, AND THE LATTER IS THROUGH PERSONAL 'EXPERIMENTATION' (I use the word lightly) AND NOT 'RESEARCH OR STUDIES' HANDED DOWN TO ME BY A WHITE COAT IN A LAB! WHAT IS IREFUTABLE IS THAT ALL I'VE ACHIEVED IN MY LIFE, I DID MYSELF, FROM EIGHT YEARS ONWARD; I'VE SELDOM HAD EVEN MINIMAL SUPPORT AND WITHIN THE SPORTING FRONT I NEVER HAD A COACH OR A SUPPORT TEAM – IT WAS ALL ME, SO I HAD TO LEARN QUICK AND THOROUGH, OR WASTE A LOT OF TIME I DIDN'T HAVE! FINALLY, I STILL FIND EVEN THE THOUGHT OF AUTHORING BOOKS, AND THIS IS MY THIRD (OR EVEN FIFTH) MAKES ME FEEL SOMEHOW UNEASY, NO-ONE EVEN IN WIDDRINGTON (AND I'VE BEEN HERE FOR 70 YEARS) KNOWS WHO I AM – I AM THE MOST ORDINARY PERSON I KNOW, NOT BETTER OR WORSE THAN ANYONE ELSE, JUST ME, AND I HOPE THAT WITHIN THE ALMOST UNIQUE PAGES THAT FOLLOW YOU MAY FIND SOMETHING AT LEAST A BIT INTERESTING.

CONTENTS

At long last, I'd like to dedicate this book to the special women in my life:

Jennifer, Mother, Linda, Julie, Nanna, Granny, Agnes,
Sybil, Sarah, Gillian, Sally and Misty!

Bet, with a shake of your heads you are all still trying to figure me out?
Stop worrying it's nearly finished – I think!

Also to

JAMES, DAVID, DAN, MICHAEL and CHRIS – I got so very lucky – Thank you!

Authoring Books and a brief personal intro!

I write the way I feel, it's deceitful as well as potentially boring not to, I'd rather not come across as a person I'm clearly not, after all, books of this nature are non-fiction and therefore based on a large element of both perceived truth as well as fact. Just as I'm not gifted enough to run with the elegance of Steve Ovett or Seb Coe, or ride with the panache and style of the Yellow Jersey, nor am I intelligent enough to copy other people's literary work, writing styles, or even content, as such the same words I use verbally are simply transferred on to paper in the very same manner as the words exit my mouth. In a free society, built on democracy, my basic rationale is simple: if you *think it*, then *say it*, and if you are bold enough to *say it*, then why not write a book and *print it*. I figure that because we don't all talk the same way then the written word should also be different and reflect the person you are – our views are what make us different, it's the differences that make us potentially less boring or more interesting; not better, I hasten to add but – well – 'different'! The Beatles were initially different as were the Stones and so was Spike, Davy Hudson and Keithie Henderson and Little Walter! Some may muse over the latter, but it's my belief that recording our thoughts in a written format should be as unique and different as our personal identity.

There is little to ponder about in my writing style, it's basic, I see myself as a very raw and untrained author and I consider that as a great place to be because it's a potentially new, untrodden world I tread with few inhibitions or rules to follow, in the latter regard I'm a loose cannon if you like, who is bound to make unapologetic statements, and unintended mistakes. Regardless, this is the third book I have written, and I've somehow managed to type every single word of all three books myself whilst taking no advice on how best a book should be written or how it should visibly appear, every word has my hidden signature attached to it, it's all just me and therefore the written word is simply my interpretation of the subjects I enthusiastically engage in! Now in contrast, 'proper skilled' authors, and those often referred to as 'ghost writers', that's those who are employed to write books for others, those 'others' who presumably can't be bothered or haven't the enthusiasm to write their own, as such employ presumed skilled people to write for them on the basis that the latter professionals are deemed as both intelligent and specifically educated, ensuring the finished article will presumably have so much more finesse and less in the way of error than an ordinary bloke like myself. I'm currently 70 years old, a bloke who left school 55 years ago at the tender age of 15 with nothing of note apart from a young, healthy, fit body, a broad, childish smile, and an outlook energised with so much immature excitement, just so pleased to be free from ink-wells, names carved callously on old wooden desks, and a few untidy exercise books. I can't remember having any fears or apprehension about an uncertain and undefined future, a future that could take me anywhere! Now, reflecting briefly on the latter statement, shortly after leaving school I almost immediately joined the Royal Navy, did it all by myself way back then, beginning by catching a morning train from the quiet of Widdrington's countrified Station to the hustling-bustling Geordie capital of Newcastle, alighting the train there I crossed the road and entered Gunner House with the infantile perceived vision of a job that would allow me to see the world on the cheap for no monetary outlay, a world that I'd imagined long ago had all blue seas married up to white seagulls surfing effortlessly on blue cloudless skies AND with the very real added bonus of a 'girl waiting just for me in every port across the globe'! Surely I'd be at the back of a lengthy queue to enlist I must have thought, regardless if there had been a queue I'd have been prepared to wait! It was all my vision, my choice, and ultimately my decision, yet just five short years earlier I was only 10 years old, still in short second-hand pants playing footy, birds nesting, and gathering rosehips, blackberries and conkers around my local woods and hedgerows surrounding Widdrington! Back to 1967 and my views then must have been similar to those which had me volunteering to enter a Secondary Boarding School for two years to finish off the remainder of my education, a unique little school consisting of wooden sheds situated in the wilds of the beautiful county of Northumberland many miles away from the comforts and security of home and family. Who wouldn't want to come with me again this time on a far greater jolly? Too good an opportunity to miss surely; however, rather surprisingly it seems no-one dreamed as I did back then and so I went to sign on to the *life on the ocean waves* all alone! Certainly beats an apprenticeship at the pit, or so it must have seemed then in the cold month of January 1967, to a 15 year old laddie, a kid so immature that he wouldn't need to start shaving for at least another four or five years, although to save face in front of my more mature colleagues I'd often follow suit, cover my face in shaving foam and just pretend while using a bladeless razor! So much for a roughie-toughie Royal Marine Commando, eh, but don't let the latter sway you too much because even in my youth I was tough, resilient and probably above all robust, I could fight my own battles, and always did!

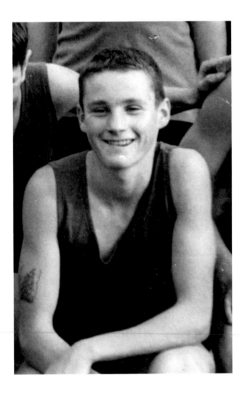

15 years of age, very fit and very healthy

Now then, leap a long way forward from that station platform in 1967, land on turf in 2021 and here I am pretty much the same excited dreamer I was back then and with a hint of *'show me the boy and I'll show you the man'*, I now write books, can you believe it? Same principle as 1967, I thought I could and there's no reason why I shouldn't, and so I do! Looking back again and for some reason, or so it seems I've gone full circle, I actually 'want' to write now; and money still, as always, has little relevance, it never did really, as such bank notes provide no motivation. What a change though, for in my earlier years at both Boarding School and the armed forces, writing just one 'solitary letter' home 'annually' was more painful than having your pecker caught in your trouser zip, with loads of 'good intentional' people hovering around saying – 'here let me help' – argh!!

The nature of my books all derive from countless vivid memories of a very active and varied life, and fortunately as far as sporting issues are concerned I have gathered a huge collection (a lifetime's) of self-penned sporting diaries, filled in daily for around 50 years, all of which are a constant reminder of who I was particularly in the sporting world, who I strove to be, who I developed into, as well as who I am now in 2021. And so, apart from my continued athletic life, I write books now and they are a real challenge and a lot of trial and error, yet I write them with the same mass of raw enthusiasm that I'd always put into both my sporting life and my working career; none of the latter was a job, it was all so much more important than that.

Now based on the above hastily written words, which includes a very short personal intro, what I'm basically saying is that any of us can write an autobiographical book – after all we've all had differing lives – but if you choose to write, take a tip from a real amateur, *'make the book your own, not a carbon copy of someone else's'*. Based on what I've written here, and you may know this already, and not for the first time, I'm struggling to say what I mean, I know what I want to say as an opener to this book, but just can't find the words I seek to express it. Maybe I am trying to make early excuses for any shortcomings in my writings! **So *try this:***

Ever heard of a band from the 1960s called the Kingsmen? They sang a song called Louie Louie in 1963! Now that *very basic* recording still, all these years later, fills me with all sorts of chills and excitement, for me it's adrenalin on tap, and the tap is turned on fully right up to number 10 on the dial, that's 10 out of 10 resulting in sheer simple youthful joy! The song is so uncomplicated, fresh, rough at the edges and above all simple, so juvenile, and the way they play it is simply 'them' because there is no pretence, no finely tuned dancing, smiling boy-band act, it's not got the panache of The Dark Side of The Moon nor does it have the musical brilliance of Sgt Peppers and if Louie Louie were played with the same musical expertise as Pink Floyd and the Beatles who recorded those two landmark latter albums, well, they'd ruin Louie Louie, perhaps it would become just too musically good – and Louie Louie is good because it's basic, even flawed, but it's them. When I close my eyes and listen to the Kingsmen playing Louie Louie, I see, in my mind's eye, five budding teenage raw musicians in cheap jeans and trainers getting a big kick out of just 'trying' – now, after all that rubbish, if you haven't guessed, what I'm trying to say is that writing a book can be the same, it doesn't have to be word perfect, it doesn't have to ooze literal brilliance, you're not trying to show the world how intelligent or accomplished you are as an 'author', the book is simply identifying *a you and a me* and aren't we just so different? Course we are! As for me, I've no A levels, no University degrees or scholarly honours, but I'm an author of a book and although there are billions of others out there, they aren't like mine – or yours if you choose to write one. I start with an empty sheet of A4 paper and a few scribbled notes, nothing copied, no discussion with anyone, just a vision.

Now, very few people are likely to read any of this, which I find, in an immature way, very reassuring; however, if you haven't worked it out let me say one more time, I see my writing as similar to that amateur musical performance by the Kingsmen, not musically fabulous I hasten to add, but rather a basic attempt to tell a story in my own individual and natural way, just having a go in the only way I know how!

Before moving on, here's a great opportunity for me to briefly pay a small personal tribute to someone I knew many, many years ago, an inspirational and motivational mentor you'll never have heard of!

A very small tribute to Sgt Marcus (Doc) Halliday P T I Royal Marine! Last seen in 1968!

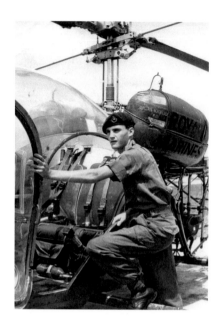

During my Royal Marine's service, I spent my life very quickly changing from uniform to shorts and vest, and just as quickly back to uniform – great fun but hectic!

I first met Doc in 1968, I was a Junior Marine in training and he was outside my room at Deal one night noisily breaking up snow-skis by stamping on them with extreme force. In the corner were several rifles used for Biathlons (skiing/ shooting competitions) with elaborate specialist sights attached to the barrels. Junior Marines were the lowest of the low (little more than hardy school kids), more so if you were the latest intake into the Depot, as far as rank and file goes we were lower than a 'worm's willie', and that's low – you spoke to others when spoken to while standing up-right to attention, and only when they asked you a question first. A short while later, somehow Doc found out that myself and Tommy Gunning and one or two others were decent runners and were big style into sport; amazingly he approached us one day and invited us to run with him, and so we'd run from Deal over to the white cliffs of Dover and back – 'freedom'! Doc was a man before his time; his knowledge on all things sporting was immense, being a British international sportsman in various sports, as well as an old style adventurer seemingly having no real superiors to answer to.

By sheer coincidence, a few days ago I dug out a letter Doc sent me in 1970 while I was in Singapore – I hoard everything; on a similar note, I still have letters written by local athlete and Commonwealth Games Marathon Champion Jim Alder who sent me similar correspondence in 1967 – anyhow, as mentioned, Doc had sent me a letter while I was in Singapore, six pages explaining the value of certain types of training, as well as advice (which wasn't fashionable then) on healthy eating etc – remember this is 1970.

What Doc told me in that letter on the 6th December 1970 is the bedrock of much that is written in this book, the test of time has shown he was right then, and although there is much water under the bridge, he is still right today on the 1st September 2021. There was nothing complex in his letter, it was all readable and made sound sense then as it still does – KEEP IT SIMPLE, and don't complicate a relatively simple subject, above all speak in a language that people understand!!

Despite us all being fundamentally different in so many ways, almost everything we do in life from birth to death is copied; from an early age we are conditioned to follow, with a silent 'keep in line' command being the accepted directive, even when there are potentially so many other pathways to choose from it seems it's so much safer to tread on ground where others have already tread, rather than be a bit more adventurous and self-determinate!

We have been bombarded for years with never-ending catalogues of fitness and health possibilities, all portrayed by either slightly overweight physicians in suits or white laboratory coats carrying laptops, folders, files, Tablets, as well as the very clever 'do everything sports watches' hanging from lapels. Others who try to guide us are a million or so apparently super fit and glowingly healthy 'looking' celebrities, models and fitness gods and goddesses with bodies that millions seemingly dream about owning. As I write and simply at random there is a magazine photo in front of me extolling the positives of yoga, the model is standing on one leg with the other at right angles resting on the opposite knee (similar to Ian Anderson's flute playing stance in Jethro Tull), both arms are directed upwards into the blue cloudless sky with an added visual bonus of the clear green ocean only feet away. At other times there are young fitness 'experts' leaping in all manners around sitting rooms, inviting ordinary non-athletic types to join in and get fit – occasionally with a promise that it can been all be achieved in just 15 minutes a day! Then there are the repeat adverts showing the carefully selected leotard-entombed model riding an expensive indoor bike soaked in sweat at a rate of knots that beggars belief, while still having the wherewithal to smile serenely at the camera. Despite all those adverts and numerous articles, two thirds of the nation, we are told, are by all accounts overweight, many are obese and there are approximately seven million of us with type two diabetes, as the incidents of heart attacks and strokes are still on the rise. I wonder how many ordinary people look at the slim-line 'athlete' performing effortlessly on the television screen before they quickly turn away terrified at the thought of such an exaggerated fitness regime, instead of being just a little inspired to at least give it a try!

If you want to encourage people into a healthy life style which includes 'regular' exercise, my view is it has to appeal to the millions of 'everyday' people, people whose lifestyles are at least similar to your own in terms of everyday living. In Doc Halliday's letter from 1970, everything he said then is still sound 50 years later; I wonder how people in 50 years' time will view the current mountains of advice given ad hoc today by the thousands who simply copy the views and books of others? *Sgt Halliday's advice is as relevant now as it was then and that's because of its simplicity, not its complexity.*

A lot of what follows, although extremely varied, is based on using myself as the proverbial Guinea pig, a lot of trial and error, that's stuff that worked for me and apparently still does! However, and this is really important, there is a big difference between being ordinary in terms of normal living and balancing everyday responsibilities whilst taking additional steps to remain active and healthy, and the life of a dedicated driven athlete – the content of the menu is the same, but, 'you' choose from it (in terms of what type and how much) what is applicable for you the individual; in other words you 'cut your cloth' as the saying goes to suit your very personal circumstances!

*To **Louise Morton**: Similar perhaps to the last mile of the marathon, writing a fairly lengthy book can towards the end become an arduous and tough experience – and your expertise and cheerful persona made the last mile of this book much more bearable. And my sincere thanks, Louise!*

Then and Now

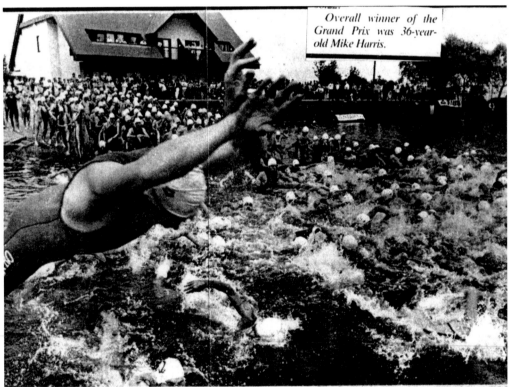

Overall winner of the Grand Prix was 36-year-old Mike Harris.

)ne competitor jumps the gun at the start of Sunday's triathlon. Picture: PETER ORM

'Exciting or what? The start of another event I went on to win, no wonder I could never find sleep afterwards, lying wide awake and buzzing with adrenalin still gushing through my veins through the dark night – and that, despite the unavoidable fatigue!'

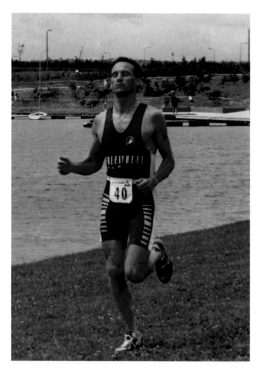

Two hours later from absolute mayhem, to a brief moment of solitude and relief

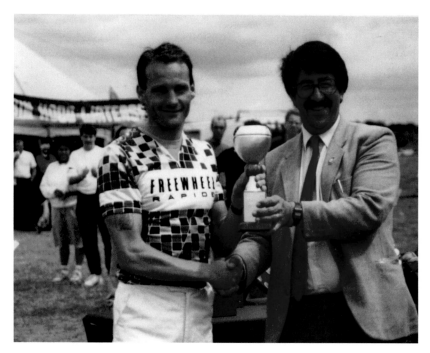

Victor takes the spoils!

Triathlon de Nice : toujou

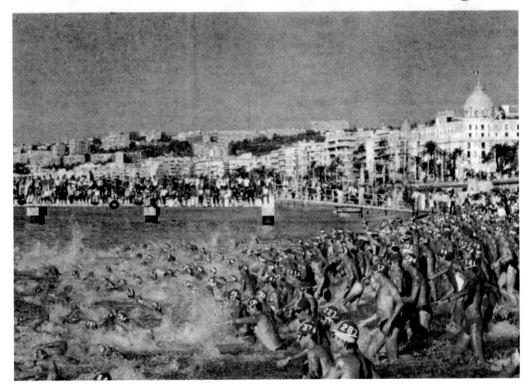

The Nice World Championships, placed 14th (First amateur)

I travelled from the North Eastern former 'pit' village of cloudy Widdrington for this event on the exotic Cote d'Azur, which shows a typical start scene from the 1984 World Championships in sunny Nice (spot the 'pale', anaemic-looking guy who was soon to lose all his 'fake tan' in the waters of the warm Mediterranean). If the start looks rough, the thousands of stinging 'jelly-fish' that accompanied us around the 3000metre swim were even more hostile, but that's the French for you, eh?

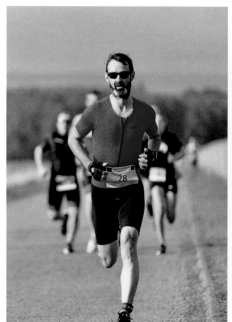 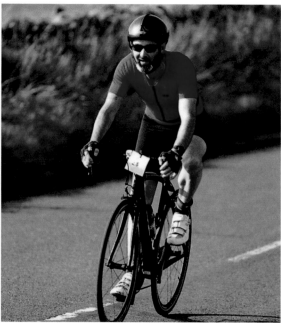

Excuse me, but this is just too fortuitous to miss, and it's just happened!

My eldest son James mentioned, out of the blue, a short while back that he'd entered a Duathlon (run 5k/bike 20k/run 2.5k). He hadn't competed in any sport since school days, so a bit of a shock, although he has always looked after himself physically. Keeping it all so very brief but on the same theme as we have been talking regarding 'amateur' sport, here is the epitome of amateur sport and the amateur athlete: James is 39 years old, like many he works 12-hour shifts, has a young family, has but one solitary bike for all occasions, and one pair of average wheels which came with the bike, one pair of soiled scruffy cycling shoes, one pair of well-worn trainers, a cycling helmet I gave him, and the cheapest tri-suit in the world (it's probably in the Guinness Book of Records); he turned up, a bit nervous and quietly without any fuss or hoorays won the event!! So proud, son, as I would have been even if you'd been last! All your own efforts – terrific!! All done on a small budget befitting the amateur athlete you are!

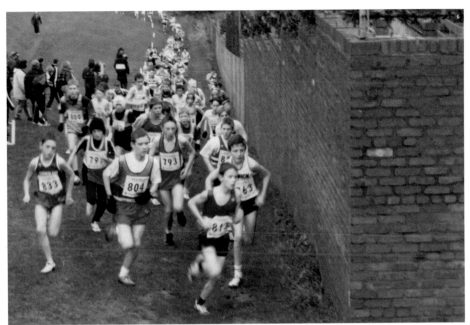

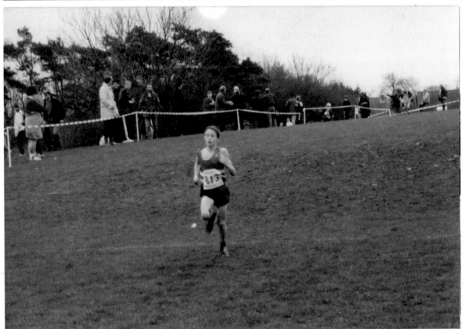

*Keeping it breifly within the family, my youngest son David
was a classy and gutsy young athlete. Here he is leading the
pack, he won several titles on both track and country.*

Hurry up, Mam, I'm going to be late!

Here's a little secret that rarely gets any airing, past or present! Both my sons were born with a rare genetic skin condition inherited from my wife's side! Called epidermis bullosa (simplex) which in brief layperson's terms means their feet blister badly, especially in warm and hot weather. It's not unusual for both my sons, and now my grandson Dan, to have several blisters on each foot. All three are tough lads and just get on with it. My sons are on their feet all day in their occupational employment, so you can only imagine the discomfort the two of them go through. The above mini-heading came straight from the mouth of my grandson Daniel whilst I was sitting watching him getting his blisters burst by Julie, his mother, before going to school.

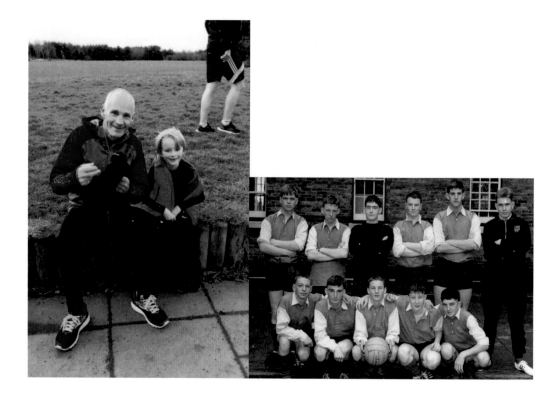

On the 2nd of November 2019, six year old Dan ran his first park run without stopping, marvellous! However, like his Grandad at that age, he enjoys football more.

How it was, and how it is (been there for many years competing – still here and still competing! (Who said 'God loves a trier'?)

Books of this nature (and this is my third), which cover many years of detail, can be viewed as an accurate and valuable *historical document* which allow the reader to make comparisons between the past and the present – simply put, looking back at how things used to be many years ago in my case from 1951, and right up to now in 2021, and then contrasting those years with the current norm can be engaging for interested parties.

I am old enough to actually remember a time when top athletes actually went to work every day, came home at the end of the day and then went training. On completion of the working week those who were athletes competed at weekends for no monetary rewards or any meaningful financial support, if the athletes then went on to win (or place) in predetermined competitions they were selected on merit before going on to represent their home nations or GB in the major games. In total contrast to athletes who at one time worked for a living, and following on from the highly successful 2020 Olympic Games in Japan where we won so many medals we could hardly keep count, and today (1/9/21) the GB Paralympic team are standing at 2nd place in the medals table with a total of 80 medals, 29 of which are gold, only China are more 'successful', even the mighty USA are 17 adrift of us, and there's another day or two to go so it's a 'certainty' we'll be get some more!* In a timely manner, while still celebrating the monumental success of the current games, the government has just announced that there will be another £232,000,000 made available to assist the current and the next sporting 'stars' to win even more medals at the next games in just three years' time. Some of the more eye-catching stars are by all accounts earning serious additional amounts of money from, amongst others, their personal sponsors. In football, and leading up to the transfer deadline, the top five Premier League teams have between them spent £523,000,000 on transfers; by contrast, the bottom five teams (in the same league) have spent 'just' £137,000,000 on transfers, a staggering discrepancy of £386,000,000 less than their affluent fellow league teams at the top end. As such, and with a degree of certainty, guess who's going to be top of the league again next year and who's going to be right at the bottom again? Money clearly creates winners! The wealthy win, the not so wealthy clearly take part but struggle! There is little guesswork needed to find sporting winners, even before a ball has been kicked, the engine has been fired, the umpire has been seated, the horse has been saddled, the boat is lowered, or the Olympians have boarded the aircraft. Football, Olympic athletes, Tennis, F1, Equestrian, Cycling, Rowing (normally) and even my sport of Triathlon are some of those who reap the rewards of generosity. What I'm saying is that sport at the so called 'top level' is simply BUSINESS and WINNING AT ALL COSTS has replaced all the interesting uncertainties that once had us all just wondering at the possibilities! Sport created to be played on a level playing field was, to a degree, built on intrigue and the unpredictable. * I was right, a couple of days ago I commented that we were currently lying 2nd in the Paralympic medals league with 80 medals, today we are up to 124 and 41 golds – bah! **I've set myself up here with what follows, which is a *'now and then'* comparison!**

In terms of athletic performance, one of the most fulfilling achievements for me as the amateur athlete I was, was the taking of seven or eight months of consistent, intensive, everyday, specifically designed training and racing every year beginning in the cold austere winter months of December or January and then seeing it all gradually build into a crescendo later that year before coming to fruition on a pre-determined solitary day in maybe June, July, August or September, culminating with an occasional big British Championship win on that one isolated day that really mattered within the athletic year. On hindsight and looking back, there is no doubt about it, I was extremely good at getting a specific performance right *on that one day that mattered*, mentally as well as physically. In truth, I had little time to sit around worrying about a forthcoming race, so busy was my life governed as it was by 40 hour working weeks. I was successful many times in events that were important to me, having won 18 British Championship medals as well as some in Europe, but looking back I was so different from most of those at the top level, because I was and indeed still am a lone-wolf, an unknown amateur athlete who had received no guidance from anyone; as such I had absolutely no support team, unlike many others who it seems 'need' people around them, I actually prospered by isolation and a huge amount of personal endeavour. Unlike the pros of today, I received absolutely no recognition for my results, although perhaps it would have been there had I gone looking for it. The only apathy attached to my athletic success was an unwillingness (a can't be bothered attitude) to seek publicity, or applause, and the latter inactivity was probably due simply to a lack of both motivation as well as available time. Being the working amateur I was, no sooner had I crossed those countless finishing lines than I was straight back to work as a 40 hour working week beckoned! I have never been unemployed and never been seriously ill, therefore I was never idle and away from work through sickness! Maybe, you can now see just why over the past five or so years I have been self-lured into writing a book or two. To be honest, although the books 'may' be interesting for some family members who follow on from me a few years from now, the books are really a bit selfish and are here for me to occasionally reflect back on when I am very old and potentially a little lonely as the world moves on leaving me in its wake, just another quiet inauspicious elderly has-been; so as I sit and reminisce, the books may be a timely reminder of what I did with my life and more importantly perhaps they may even make me smile in some sort of very quiet self-appreciation way!

Returning to the theme, 'then and now', harbouring many months of training and storing the physical gains within the unique athletic body of the individual, before releasing those gains and capitalising on all the work on a specifically intended day, whilst additionally competing against hundreds of other equally fit and determined athletes, is a culmination of many skills, with the addition of a little luck, that hard to define little word which is so often the difference between winning and being runner-up!

Living in the remote non-athletic backwater of the North East, I did many 50mph boring creeping along the motorway journeys in a wreck of an unreliable vehicle to compete 'doon sooth' against the rest and best of this country's athletes. For this event, I travelled alone on this occasion setting off before the sun rose at 3am. More often than not with Jennifer riding 'shot-gun' and the lads crammed up together in the back (I said NO to the dog – harsh I know, but he smelt 'orrible!) would travel with me, with the lads competing to see who could poop the loudest, as Jennifer unperturbed by the ongoing competition, hummed an obscure unknown song as she does, and read her romantic novel as I listened to some annoyingly unfashionable R n B. It's fair to say, we must have been a somewhat strange ensemble of a family – bet the Taliban wouldn't detain us for long before they'd let us go, eh? As the boys waved enthusiastically from the rear window! Back to the day in question, and there was a huge field of several hundred competitors from every corner of the UK with us all diving into the lake together. Although I was 37 then, I was in great form, having won the British Championships a short while previously and was on a very successful run culminating in several big nationwide wins, which would go on for a while yet. Anyhow, I eventually won the event by more than two minutes and on conclusion while clutching another trophy, I travelled back up North chewing on some fast-decaying, sun-hardened, pre-prepared cheese and tomato sandwiches, all swilled down with the warm cloudy remnants of my bike's competition water bottle! Arriving home stiff and tired, I'd empty the car first before having a shower and then gorge heartily on a wonderful plain but very welcome homemade basic meal, after which, as usual, I'd go to bed and sleep very badly if at all, which was/is the norm, before I'd roll out of bed at 6am to begin my next working day beginning with my compulsory swim in Ashington's 25 yard pool, before travelling to my place of work at Ponteland and the very different challenge of training up a workforce of 5000 – just another 40-hour working week, one of 52, while somehow still managing to combine as always three times a day training aimed at the next weekend's competition!

Going back to the title of this early chapter and the contrasting theme of *'then and now',* and currently our athletes and their considerable entourage of specialist helpers have just returned from the Olympics in Japan, millions of monetary pounds lighter, but much heavier in terms of medals, and in absolute heroic glory (apparently even 'inspiring' her majesty the Queen, not BMX Ma'am surely?). Accompanying the adulation fit for heroes are the ever present interviews which continue to repeatedly extol the brilliance of the athletes as well as the common ever-present mantra of *'all the sacrifices'* they've made in their journey to represent Team GB in the holy grail of sporting events which is the Olympic Games, while collecting the ever-growing numbers of medals. The wonderfully successful Paralympians will soon be home to join the other GB athletes and will wallow in the magnitude of their success and rightly so; regardless, there are some successful medallists I now genuinely feel a bit sorry for and that's because once upon a time when things were 'equal' in the sporting world, much like other similar nations to us, 'our' medallists were a rarity, as such most of those who brought a medal home were very special because we didn't accumulate that many then and the small amount of athletes who did triumph were unusual as well as special and therefore rightly revered. Now in 2021 here we are with so many numerous victors (which has become the absolute norm) all chewing happily on their newly attained and well-earned medals for the photos (I've never understood that gesture, is there a meaning behind biting into a medal for a photo?), many successful athletes now get lost in the growing expanding throng and league of fame due to the swell of gold, silver and bronze!! The current rise of sporting stars is not dissimilar perhaps to the masses of ever-expanding numbers of celebs as such few individuals now stand out as they once did because they're becoming as common as the sound of the everyday angry screams of *'resign'* emanating across the benches at Westminster!! Once the adulation has receded, as sure as night follows day, out will come a multitude of biographies depicting lives seemingly so very different from the rest of us; it seems that to be a star, sporting or otherwise, it is an absolute necessity to have had a Dickensian-type childhood built around struggle, racism, strife, sexism, bullying and poverty! The stars have very few 'happy' autobiographies – clearly they sell better and are more eye-catching in the newspaper serialisations if there is a boat-load of grief, sadness, bullying, mental health issues and controversy of any sort! Oh well, on reflection the rest of us ordinary people have clearly been extremely lucky even if in certain circles we'd probably be seen as a bit boring!!! Being ordinary does have its advantages, although it clearly doesn't pay as well!

And so, in contrast to the way triathlons were then, in 2021 all the big championship events around the world have far fewer athletes, resulting in a rather tame spectacular of around 30 or so wonderful athletes politely lining up on a pontoon or jetty with a yard's space between each competitor before the Caxton sounds and they all dive in unison into clear transparent water. Ha! 'In my day' there were often hundreds of us stood around at a lakeside picking our noses (getting colder by the minute), or a similar waterfront (as depicted here on the wonderful French Riviera) which resembled a chaotic scene perhaps not dissimilar to match day at St James' Park 30 minutes before a Toon home game, pushing and jostling as we waited for the anticipated 'gun' and if the starting gun didn't sound soon enough a competitor would accidentally pre-empt with an unintended cough, flinch, fart or sneeze and with a comment of *'was that it?'* and with a nod, we'd be off – no stopping us, mad, mad people, identities hidden by swim caps and goggles, the idiots like me were at the front fighting, the intelligent at the back complaining of a headache or wrong time of the month. False start or not, we were too powerful; as such we wouldn't be coming back to try again and calamity would rein for a while till the bunch sorted itself out and became gradually smaller and consequently more orderly. Currently, having left the water in Transition 1, the pros now take on the cycle section by going round and round in a big almost orderly bunch circling for several laps, following in the slipstream of the leader with little change in positions. In contrast, we would exit the water and the bike transition park after the swim and disappear for 25 or 30 miles into the undulating varied countryside before straggling back in in ones, twos, or threes to Transition 2 with huge gaps having developed between the best triathletes and the rest as the gaps continued to grow, as we'd contest the 10k run which would finally sort out the overall positions. *Now which event would you rather watch?*

If you want 'entertainment' in sport, I'd advise you to watch *'amateur '* sport more, and by comparison it's dirt cheap with no entry fees, hot-dogs *two a penny*! Amateur triathlons are much the same now as they were , except for the inclusion of wetsuits and attractive clothing attire, mass starts, with big and varied fields are still prevalent with competitors always coming and going, and transitions are a lively hive of activity, with quite large scale on-going changes in positions. The venues are also often user and spectator friendly. A lot of people smile at 'people events', particularly at the end because everyone has a personal story (mainly about the bad luck that always follows them around!), and win or lose, it isn't a 'business', it's all just intended as a challenge and that's maintained – but it's also fun. Harriers League events are similar, as are Park Runs, there is little in the way of prizes, hence most people young and not so young are there for the personal challenge, regardless at the end, little sleep is lost following a below-par performance because it's not business. In contrast with professional sport, where we know with a degree of certainty who is likely to win, especially in F1, Tennis, Triathlon, Football and several other 'well heeled' sports, as money continues to speak and so often makes the difference between the affluent winning and the much poorer losing.

Having said all the latter, many, but by no means all, of current day athletes and sporting celebrities are role models, despite the massive support, no-one can do the work and preparation for you and not all can cope with the very real mental anxiety and tension that comes with high expectations – with a bit of genuine envy, my hat goes off to you. **Talking of amateur sport!**

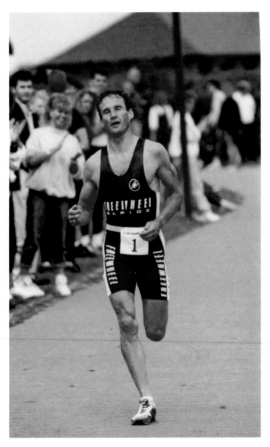

You could still win events as an amateur, in my day!
A British championship win at Milton Keynes.

> **"People are able to wonder at the height of mountains and the huge waves of the sea, the vast compass of the ocean, the circular motion of the stars and then pass by themselves without wondering at all"**

St Augustine said that – were you there, Grandad?
No, son, I was on my bike, Ossie told me!

HEALTH (WHY BOTHER?)

If you were asked a question in an intelligence test, 'within a league of priorities and on a scale of 1-10, where would you put the importance of health?', presumably, for the purpose of attaining high marks, the astute, logical person would place it close to the top, if not at the very top. Why? Because arguably without good health you have nothing! I mean, is a million pounds worth a million pounds if you are dying of self-inflicted heart disease? Or is a nice big lump sum and the assurance of a monthly pension worth anything at all if you are not well enough to spend it?

It could be argued that everything we have done in the past, everything we do now, and everything we do in the future quite literally revolves around our past, current and future health. The unhealthier we are or the less fit we become, the greater the self-imposed limitations will be – and that's a fact.

If good health could be bought, we would all fork-out a sum and buy it – no question! Why then are we so willing to give it away? Presumably we would all lay claim to being sane, yet only a lunatic would want a sick or unhealthy body.

Good health is a gift that most of us are lucky to be born with, but it can be a temporary gift. Most of us take it for granted; rarely think about it perhaps, until, that is, something goes wrong. Similarly, perhaps we may rarely give much thought to our teeth until we get a touch of toothache then it's 'just let me check that toothbrush again'. Prevention has got to be better than cure (especially when you consider the current demand and strain on the NHS).

The body is truly a work of art and that's not an exaggeration. With a billion pounds you couldn't build one, and we're all different. We are the most complex thing on this planet, you and I. The complexity of a human being is beyond comprehension to me; the more you ponder it – the greater the miracle of it expands. It is a continuous automatic process of change. It regulates itself in terms of growth, temperature, movement, thought, rejuvenation, pain, pleasure, energy, fatigue or whatever and is never allowed the luxury of being turned off.

The heart, for example, begins work four weeks after conception and continues without rest till we die. The average adult's (if there is such a thing) heart beats about 70 times each minute, that's about 100,000 times each day, transporting 2,000 gallons of blood around the body, enough to fill a small road tanker!

Although the physiological make-up of the body is complex, the overall maintenance of it is relatively simple. However, neglect the maintenance at your peril. I think we need to be aware of neglect and the possible consequences of it. What is abundantly clear (and rightly so) is that *your* body is *your* concern. Regardless of the job you do, you can be assured that no one else will take responsibility for it, either now or in the future, and why should they?

Assuming that health and a degree of fitness is important and worthy of some thought and attention (if only because it makes sound sense), why then don't the vast majority of us take it seriously? Maybe we are not sufficiently educated or schooled in human biology, maybe we don't have time, perhaps 'other things' are more important or could it be, simply, that we are just not motivated. *Stating 'fact' is not, in my book, being offensive! So let me be direct whilst being factual, many people are lazy and have a 'can't be bothered' attitude.* People need to be motivated, address the latter (motivation) and maybe we could redress people's priorities. I'm sure that motivation is the key factor because if we can't see a reason for something we are bound to question it, or worse still, ignore it totally.

Motivation (short term)

Being reasonably fit and healthy makes us feel good; it is reassuring and gives peace of mind; it gives credibility (especially perhaps in uniformed personnel) and creates confidence; it probably even slows down the aging process. Even within middle-age or old-age, fitness can give you the physical capacity to do just about anything.

Motivation (long term)

Personally, I have to admit to being concerned about the limitations associated with old-age and, generally people tend to equate old age with catastrophic physical decay. I fear the concept of not being self-reliant. Images of old people sitting in a circle singing 'Cushy Butterfield' does not appeal! In a nutshell, I don't want to be severely limited just because I've reached a certain age, or retirement and maybe (because there's no guarantee) if I do things right now, I'll have a better than even chance of doing ok later.

The subject of health can be as complex or as simple as required, depending on the aim of the end product. The simple side is that if we eat reasonably well, exercise occasionally and are able to laugh regularly then we are not too far away. The complex side is that we are all different. Fundamentally, we're the same, but essentially every individual has different needs depending on aim, age, gender, size, ability and even motivation. Therefore, it makes sense that each of us should give careful thought to our own individual exercise routine and dietary intake.

As you would expect, having been involved in health and fitness departments for many years, including 24 years with Northumbria Police, I'm passionate about the subject of health. I find the human body, its actions and mannerisms, absorbingly interesting. I also don't have a problem selling health and fitness to interested parties because unlike some other salesmen I've bought the product myself and I'll continue with it for as long as I'm able. So, there's no deception on my part.

However, experience has shown that extolling the virtues of health (from whatever angle) doesn't always work – invariably people will either take it on board as a 'necessity' or ditch it, as rubbish! It's a personal choice and I fully respect that.

The purpose of the remainder of this publication is designed to offer readable, non-complex advice on health and fitness, and I'll try hard to make the content both interesting and unpredictable; telling someone what aerobics means is simply repetition, it's been done before, but because it fits within the remit of a chapter I include it. At this stage it's really important for me to state that I'm not 'telling' anyone what to do – I've no right to do that; after all, it's your body – I'm simply saying this is the menu and you may want to consider the use of some of the things available on it to improve or better what you already have. So, should you feel inclined to take a more positive side to life, and improve your current health, hopefully the information herein may be of benefit. Your next move could be the biggest investment you ever make!

Concluding this early chapter, I'll add that this book, is in many ways, a one-person discussion on the subject of health and fitness, a subject I have been involved in for most of my life. The subject though is often tidal by nature, by which I mean it ebbs and it flows: one minute it is topical and many of us acknowledge its importance, but the next moment, just like the tide, it has disappeared over the horizon and is once again unfashionable and trivial. Personally, I find it difficult to understand why people can't eat 'reasonably' well – and exercise 'occasionally' – especially when it's so simple and the alternative is to eat badly and never exercise and the repercussions of the latter are potentially life changing. 'Trends' are part of the problem and trends are often engineered by an individual such as a current fashionable celebrity who sees yet another possible avenue to further promote their shrinking famous persona, and trends, just like fashions, seldom last. *A commitment to health is also a bit like the first down payment of a life insurance policy or a long term endowment; it seems, at least at the beginning, that there is no immediate identifiable gain or need, so our investment has little in the way of initial appeal. But of all the gifts we are given or we accumulate, health is the greatest gift of all. Now that's a huge statement but logic dictates and cements the choice.*

Preface and ... A starter for seventy!

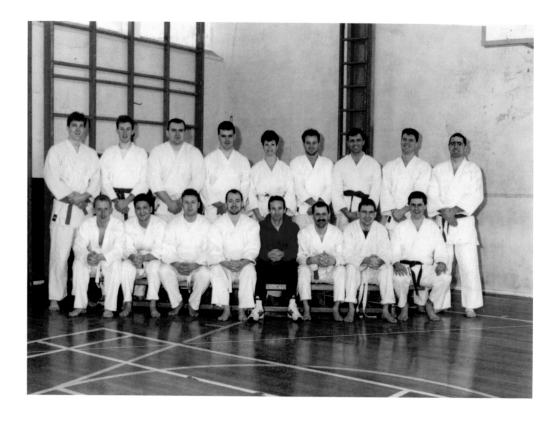

Even work was energetic, here running a two week self defence instructor course

Simply by chance, I met an old work colleague a few months ago, and as is the norm some casual smiling and humorous banter ensued. As people often do with me, it wasn't long before he asked how 'you fill your time in since retiring and now you'll be no longer training and competing'. Oh, I said casually, '*I'm still going, I've never stopped, I still train every day and look for competitions as I've always done*'. He looked pleasantly surprised, being influenced no doubt because of my obvious advancing years, before commenting that he had first met me in 1988 when he joined the police, and how I'd occasionally do the mile and a half run with his 'intake', always leading them in by a considerable margin. Now in those distant days, probationers were graded in their physical performances and for the run they were given a score whereby 9 minutes and under was classed as excellent, 9mins – 10mins was good, 10-12 was acceptable and anything over 12 was classed as poor and a re-run would be the outcome for the latter. The women got a little more time to account for gender issues. In 1988 I was British Triathlon Champion for the 3rd time training three times every day for triathlon events. Now, accelerate to 2020 at the time of this brief meeting with my former colleague and 32 years on from the '88 meeting and here I was still training regularly at least once every day but twice a day wasn't/ isn't rare. At the time of this chance meeting – and I couldn't recall his name (and that's always embarrassing but with 5000 people I was never going to remember all) – he quickly did some sums and said *so since our first meeting in 1988 you've never stopped?* That's about it, I replied, it's not clever, it's just what I do, amongst other things of course, before I added 'so, in 1988 I was 37, so here we are in 2020 and I'm 69, that's another 32 years and I'm very much the same today as I was then in 1988!' By-the-way, I was running 6 minute miles last year so I'd still be leading the groups in even today, and savouring a rated 'excellent' result even at 69!

I've been a serious self-coached 'practitioner *of physical activity*' all my life, that's from an infant of four years of age in 1955 when I had my very first competitive foot race, right up to and including today, when as a 'middle-aged' superbly fit 70 year old male athlete I have just completed yet another normal three-hour daily work out. **As the title of this book suggests, all my life has been an unintended 'physical experiment'.** I've competed at the highest levels in various sports, often in a Great Britain tracksuit, always as a loner with no support team, and always been self-coached. Now that's 66 years of immense non-stop daily physical activity which I'm hoping will give me a different and even unique level of credibility, allowing me to author this book whilst at the same time competing with all the professional physicians, models, and celebrities who have also authored a book on the current fashionable theme of health and fitness. Whilst it seems so much of the experience and expert advice offered by some others is derived and 'handed down' to them from the never ending repetitive references to *'research and studies have indicated'* – in contrast, the vast majority of my writings and observations have been acquired through decades of personal 'on the shop floor' experience whilst toying with the unremitting reality of results through *trial and error* – in other words, I'd try something till I thought I'd eventually got it as near as damn it right (based on results), or move and change direction whilst considering other possibilities. Because I'm still able to perform with distinction after all these years suggests I either got immensely lucky or, alternatively, knew what I was doing. Anyhow tomorrow's another day and I am always vigilant regarding any change in physical performance or general health, I really am very much switched on and I don't miss much. Apart from my personal experiences there is another aim with this book and that is to simply offer a 'different', non-complex, easy to read and understandable book designed specifically *'for the ordinary by the ordinary!'* (I use the word 'ordinary' as a compliment by the way – in today's celebrity-obsessed world ordinary people are a truly special and select bunch that I'm proud to belong to). Another thing: I won't talk about things I haven't any experience with, that way at least my views are honest and without guesswork.

A final comment before I move on: the views that follow are all mine and based on my life's experiences and most certainly they don't make me absolutely right, just as I can agree with some other people's comments – some of the time – I don't agree with their comments all the time – so if you're interested, please just take from the book what you will, and good luck. I hope it all makes a bit of sense (you know, I've once again personally typed every single word!) and is in some way different but with the difference perhaps making it at least 'interesting'!

A day in the life 2021! It's important, I think, to state that I train the way I do, not through vanity or even to prolong my life, I do what I do because I am still an 'athlete', it's *pride* more than anything because I like to give a good account of myself in athletic competitions, and when I stop competing, and it won't be long – then I'll ease up! What I'm saying is that I'm not at all recommending that others do what I do, there are many other ways, of course, of being fit and healthy and within this book we'll have a look at a few.

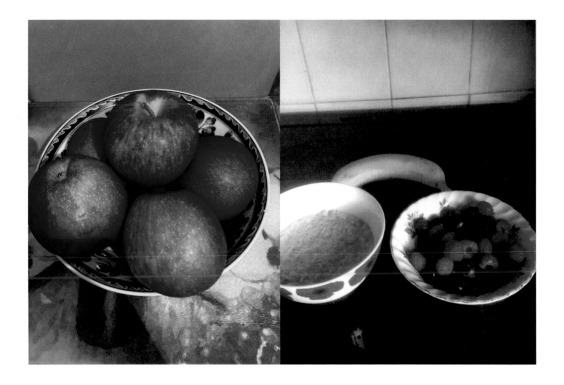

English apples are best!

Today it's Sunday the 17th January 2021, and just as with any other morning of the year, I got out of bed, dressed and grabbed an apple or two to chew on my way out to walk the beautiful Misty, our 'mature' family dog, and the two of us will meander for 45 minutes or an hour (if she's in good fettle) over the fields and woods that surround Widdrington. When we arrive back, I'll feed Misty first before making myself a bite to eat for breakfast. So I heat up a bowl of cheap Co-op porridge and whilst I'm waiting I have a couple of handfuls of rinsed blueberries, followed by a mixture of red and black grapes. After two minutes the porridge is ready and I'll sweeten it up with a chopped banana and a handful of raspberries; once consumed I'll watch the news (for as long as I can bear it) with a cup of coffee – if I am to train hard this morning my coffee is caffeinated, as it helps to mobilise a bit more energy; if the planned session is steady or easy I have de-caff. Afterwards I'll clean my teeth before riding my bike for two hours, always at a good clip, if only to stay warm in the January air, or go running for up to eight miles. I rarely exceed two hours on the bike at the moment, as to do so will probably result in a reduction of pace, and at my age quality is more important than quantity. Off the bike I'll do a bit of strength and mobility work before having a shower, and it's now around 1pm. For lunch, and depending on the effort I've given on the bike/run, I'll have either two eggs on toast (for the protein needed to re-fuel and repair my fatigued legs) or a bowl of home-made lentil soup or broth with bread or a cup of tea to follow. That's my day up to 2pm. Later I'll walk Misty again, before having an evening meal of *Geordie delight* – that's food I've eaten my entire life which used to sit comfortably within the northern working man's territory and used to fuel men working in heavy industries: porridge and fruit, potatoes and veg with either fish or maybe mince (I use Quorn regularly – can't tell the difference), hotpot, shepherd's pie, cauliflower cheese, liver and onions, egg, beans and chips etc; apart from Sunday lunch I don't tend to eat too much meat if I can help it. My wife Jennifer is a truly superb 'thrifty' cook who can turn any morsels of uneaten scraps of food into the tastiest meal you'll find anywhere; if I don't eat it all – well I get it tomorrow, and maybe even the day after that! Just as it was when I was a kid – accompanied then as it is now by a familiar repetitive comment of '*waste not want not, Michael, now get stuck in, because there's nothing else!*' I like plain food and I like plenty of it!

I've got detailed annual training diaries going back about 45 years and they're as useful now as indeed they were then, maybe even enabling me with a degree of credibility to say **'MY personal research has indicated'**, or indeed, **'MY recent trials and studies have demonstrated …!'** Today is my 105th consecutive bike ride, that's a lot of riding AND a lot of 'thinking!', the latter made possible by the self-imposed isolation that accompanies the endurance athlete. I've always trained alone, a habit going back years when time was of the essence whilst balancing three times a day training incorporated into 40 hour working weeks, as well as family responsibilities. Before cycling took hold last year, I had 77 consecutive runs (that's every day), normally between 5 and 11 miles in duration at varying speeds before (and I should have had more sense) the dreaded reoccurring Achilles* problem led me back to the bike; as always the bike's proved a blessing and I can't feel the Achilles at all whilst pedalling! **In 2020 I trained 363 days!** Within the context of this book that CONSISTENCY is a real important element as you'll see.

Already I can hear some murmuring, 'aye it's alreet if ya retired and not working', so let me say at this point the days mentioned above have been nothing other than 'normal' my entire life. As mentioned, I have approximately 45 plus annual training diaries if proof was ever needed. I trained two and three times a day for decades (before work in the morning, during my lunch break at work and then again in the evening when the day's work was over – seven days a week) whilst never being unemployed, never had so much as a single day's sick leave, or had the doctor write me a sick note; additionally for approximately 40 years I've never taken a pill or medication such as aspirin, codeine, paracetamol, cold/flu relief or whatever! In short, I suppose I'm proud that I've cost my country nothing! Never had a hospital bed (touch wood) and rarely used our local clinic. Even when competing for Great Britain for years it cost my country nothing apart from competition clothing and travelling expenses. When competing abroad for GB I occasionally (rather than embarrassingly mince up and ask the boss for special leave) took annual leave and when I returned home I was back to work within a day or two. How times change!

I got my first Achilles tendon injury (although I didn't realise it then, and we called it a 'sore' ankle) when I was running in 1964/65 and I'd be 13 or 14 years of age at boarding school, and it's been the one reoccurring injury throughout the 57 years since! Today is the 23/2/2021, and I've revisited this page with another Achilles injury picked up this morning during the last mile of a seven-mile run! Oh dear!

Bear with me please, I am currently simply writing, as if in a verbal conversation, before being stimulated enough to move on.

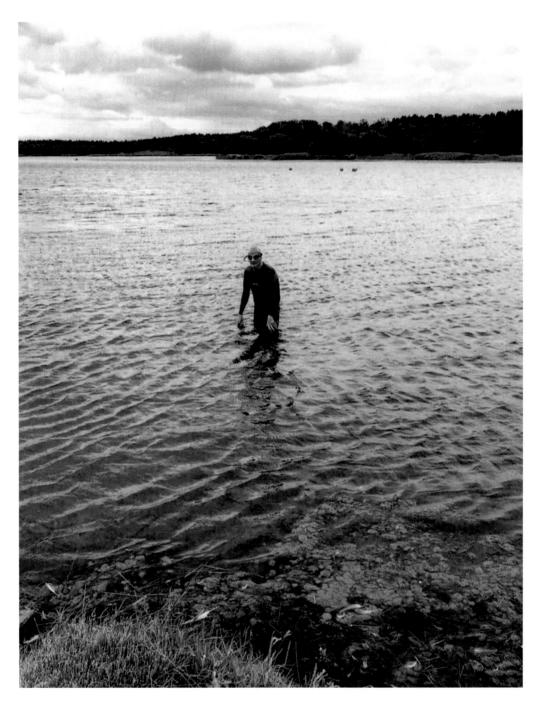

When I left the Marines, in the mid 1970s, I helped turn a colossal open-cast mud pile into the above lake – 45 years on it now resembles paradise. I regularly swim here while additionally using its pathways for triathlons and park runs.

I've often found the *beginning* of a project or the *start* of an activity the most difficult element within the whole intended process. For example, the 'beginning' of a lengthy bike ride with the threatening wind and rain hovering on the horizon, or maybe the 'thought' of a timed 'flat out' run which I know through years of experience is going to add more self-inflicted pain on my battered body and consequently hurt like hell, or what about an 'anticipated' freezing open water swim in a murky swan-infested lake with the unwelcome addition of bird droppings floating in and out of my gob, as the spooky unwelcome reeds silently reach up and tenderly caress my kicking legs. Looking back even the predictable 'commencement' of yet another classroom talk or lecture which I did over the years (and I've done thousands) were an equally uncertain and difficult part of the exercise, indeed just like the thought of getting out of bed on a mid-winter morning – **'the 'thought' of some things often exceeds the actual deed, in terms of difficulty!'** However, experience throughout many years has always shown that once I push off from the curb and 'click-in' to my pedals, or once I start my stopwatch signifying the beginning of that flat-out 'timed' run, or once I've taken that first tentative step and began the tip-toeing process into that chilly water (doing my utmost to keep my genitalia warm and cosy for just a little longer) before the cold swamps my shrinking, retreating, and condensed manhood, well, it does get easier. As mentioned, I also used to have the same uncertain reservations before delivering educational classroom sessions on a variety of specialist subjects, but once I'd confidently commenced and made eye contact with as many students as possible and given an initial verbal introduction greeting along the lines of 'good morning, how are you all, just by way of introduction my name's Mike Harris', before quickly adding 'don't believe all you may have heard about me, only some of it is true!' – well, from that point onwards, just like exercise, bear with it as it does get easier, as a mass of subject knowledge, a ton of enthusiasm, combined with a word or two of intended humour would take over a familiar and well-rehearsed personal format. And so, here we are yet again, and after much thought I've taken the first step and actually started another book, and once past the beginning and with a degree of optimism I hope that very soon the book and the ideas I envisage will begin to take a logical and readable format.

And so back to the beginning. I actually commenced writing this 'potential' book on the 11th January 2021 with an attitude of 'well you've nothing to lose, why not!'. In brief, and despite a barrage of other books appearing daily in the press, I thought the time was right for reasons I'll come to soon, and I've a host of things to share with anyone who may be tempted to open the front cover. For the most part the content is all based around my *seventy years* of what could be described as 'immense everyday physical activity' combined and partnered with a multitude of real-life experiences. As with my autobiographical books, I've no doubt this one will be nothing if not unique; after all, as mentioned, I'm 70 years old with a CV bursting with personal self-made solo achievements, and reassuringly unlike so many of the beautiful eye pleasing modern model type authors, I'm not remotely physically attractive (except perhaps to Misty our aging Labrador who simply adores me, I think?). I would also state categorically I am not interested one iota in fame and fortune and as with my other books, once written they'll receive almost no promotion. I am ordinary by anyone's observations and more than happy to be that way, as opposed to joining the thousands of anxious, self-obsessed celebrities who currently emerge from every nook and cranny with their words of wisdom designed to help us ordinary mortals out. I do, however, sincerely hope the content of the finished article here will be in some way interesting if only from the perspective of it being original, and as such very different from the numerous repetitive books on health and fitness currently saturating the post-Christmas market. Another personal reason for writing, to be brutally honest, is I have to admit to currently being 'bored rigid' with winter generally and the dull inclement weather it always brings with it; there's also the continuous repetitive morbidity hanging over the world from the Covid-19 virus, which you can't possibly escape, with the immensely sad influx of daily statistics (they even send them to me on my mobile with a 'ping' I know another's arrived – although I don't ask for them) that influence all our days and nights. And so, I've decided I need something to get my teeth into apart from my daily physical activities of walking, running, cycling or digging at my allotment, as well as an obsessive relationship with playing my guitars – now the latter hobby is for me, sheer therapy, and, it doesn't hurt!

Bluesman and sublime guitar genius Albert King once sang 'If it wasn't for bad luck, I wouldn't have no luck at all!', Bringing that lyric right up to the current 2021 he'd probably sing – 'If it wasn't for bad news, we'd have no news at all!' I'm getting ahead of myself here (I may add my own simple take on 'mental health issues later), but the media are a huge negative on us all – don't they make you miserable? News (good or bad) is news and of course I appreciate that, but the repetitive continuous current theme of morbidity is way over the top, I mean have you ever listened to the news over the past year and just once felt 'jolly' afterwards? There has to be some good news – somewhere!

To tempt me even more to write, I know this venture will do me good from another angle, and that is I'm having to use my brain on activities (writing a book) which is not normally within my comfort zone (although this isn't the first book I've authored); additionally, in the process of writing it'll refresh my rusty computer and keyboard skills. And so, as mentioned, I'll be 70 years old on the 11th August, and this 'project' will give me something different to aim for whilst speedily running up to my *three score years and ten,* and maybe if I can keep myself motivated I could get it all ready by my birthday, so my deadline for finishing it will be seven months from now, bags of time!!!

To: *Jasper Evenue Barnfather, George Fenwick Barnfather, Nicky 'the ghost' Barnfather and Robert Demery Prime Barnfather: stay out of trouble, boys and god bless, till we meet again!*

BEFORE CONTINUING!

I DON'T KNOW IF THIS IS RELEVANT – BUT I'LL SAY IT ANYHOW. IF YOU THINK THE END PRODUCT OF THIS BOOK IS UNPROFESSIONAL, OR MAYBE NOT OF THE SAME PANACHE AS OTHER MORE EDUCATED AURTHORS, YOU'RE PROBABLY RIGHT, AND I WOULDN'T DREAM OF DEFENDING MYSELF IN THE LATTER RESPECT. I WRITE MY BOOKS THE ONLY WAY I KNOW HOW, AND THAT'S LIKE HAVING A CONVERSATION WITH A FRIEND. NOW AT THE MOMENT I FEEL 'PUNCH DRUNK' BECAUSE I'M ALL OVER

THE PLACE WITH THIS BOOK, HONESTLY, IT'S A BIT LIKE HAVING A DRINK WITH MATES, ONE MINUTE YOU'RE HAVING A RELEVANT AND 'RARE' INTELLIGENT CONVERSATION, THE NEXT YOU GO FOR A PEE – AND WHEN YOU RETURN THE CONVERSATION (WHICH YOU CAN'T REMEMBER ANYHOW), HAS MOVED ON. CURRENTLY THIS BOOK IS LIKE THAT, I KEEP RETURNING TO SOME CHAPTERS BECAUSE THEY DON'T FEEL RIGHT. WHAT I MEAN IS I'VE SO MANY IDEAS BUT 'WHERE AND HOW TO INCORPORATE THEM THEM ALL?'. WHAT I DO FIND, AND IT'S LATE IN THE DAY, IS THAT AIRING YOUR THOUGHTS IN A WRITING FORMAT IS PROBABLY SIMILAR TO AIRING THE SAME THOUGHTS VERBALLY WITH A PSYCHOLOGIST – IT'S A KIND OF THERAPY, THE ONLY DIFFERENCE IS YOU DON'T BORE THE PROFESSIONAL WHO WOULD PROBABLY HAVE BEEN STIFLING YAWNS WHILST TRYING TO DISGUISE THE FACT WITH AN ATTEMPTED INTERESTED LOOK COMBINING BOTH EMPATHY AND FEIGNED INTEREST!

Today is the 24th May 2021 – I had a race yesterday, my first in the 70 plus year category and I'm currently thumbing through the earlier pages of this book again while I contemplate taking it all to the publishers soon, maybe? My legs are sore today because I had that race yesterday, a Duathlon consisting of a 2.65k run – 20k bike – and a 5.75k run. I finished 5th 'overall', a bonus as I was quite possibly the oldest person in the *race*. A nice surprise as I've so many irritating 'niggles' I almost didn't go! I was up at 5am for a start time of 7.32am and even at 5am I still wasn't sure whether to go to the event. I took the dog out for a short walk and was limping, my left Achilles was sore, I was optimistically hoping the soreness was simply down to stiffness after a night's sleep. Anyhow a glutton for punishment and with little to lose, I went. My 'game plan' was to take the first run easy/steady, then if I got through it, to bike quite hard (not flat out) and to take the first of the two remaining run laps steady; if I was still in the event then I aimed to conclude by throwing any caution to the wind with a faster last lap! It worked! Anything learnt? Yes, you are never through with learning, you must always be ready to adjust to suit the occasion, *and for me the bonus was yet again, that it's better to try and maybe lose, rather than not try at all, and 'wonder!'.*

HEALTH AND FITNESS BOOKS – THERE'S THE REAL ONES AND THE MAKE-BELIEVE COPIED ONES!

Just a thought to kickstart this chapter! I wonder how I'd be received if having read a book on *health and fitness*, I then take the information straight from within the covers of that book and turn the detail into yet 'another' Health and Fitness book? In the process of doing that I quietly remove the original author's name and replace theirs with mine. Would I, could I, get away with it? The answer of course is an absolute yes, and it seems to happen all the time; few things are original these days. Following on from that; furthermore, to encourage a preponderance of readers I also 'alter' my 'less than attractive face' and manufacture a new much more presentable front, I do that by the application of a mass of cosmetics – professionally applied, of course, now the latter 'make-up' of course it has to be said, is not a genuine 'mirror image' of my current self, nevertheless and reassuringly it instantly succeeds in ridding me of the age induced wrinkles I have mysteriously accumulated over the years and turns my sun and weather beaten skin (befitting a 70-year-old athlete), into an unrecognisable Adonis of a man. My face is now resplendent and just oozes health, as I'm transported centre stage from sitting room to the front cover of 'my' new book. I have now made a miraculous journey and with more than a little help I have transferred from the knowledgeable 70-year-old into a very attractive 30-year-old, good looking and youthful young man who makes you go weak at the knees, mmm mm! Once sufficiently 'doctored' (altered) by whatever it takes, my new face acts as the final motivator to the potential buyer – *'whatever he's on, I want some!'*, resonates! Once again, would I get away with the 'mask'? Or would I be ridiculed (not just by my intrigued mates and family or Jennifer's bathroom shaving mirror) before being sectioned and put away in secure accommodation – till I 'got better'!

Yet at the time of writing this book, it seems almost anyone who dares to shave their body and wear an eye-catching leotard or a skin-tight pair of silk shorts with not a solitary body hair in sight, accompanied by a mountain of facial cosmetics, as well as the purchased expensive new eye catching, 'must have obligatory', brilliant dulux-white gleaming teeth can author a book on Health and Fitness. Finally, as a last gesture, the vision of loveliness is partnered with a few well-chosen introductory words and a quote such as – *'I promise you, this book will change your life'* – or *'here's a brand new miracle physical workout programme that's guaranteed to change your life in as little as 30 minutes!'* Caught up in the mystique and at least intrigued, the ever optimistic punter opens the book to find activities, not as expected from the mountains and meadows of Kathmandu, but rather straight from the school pupils' Physical Exercise GCSE guide, and yes there they are again – the obligatory press-ups, leg raises, ab crunches, dips and a few other time-in-memorial exercises that people were doing centuries ago, even before the Roman leader Hadrian laid a brick at Wallsend. The sting is finally complete, and the would-be athlete places their well-earned dosh on the counter, and leaves the booksellers with a smile, while muttering '30 minutes eh'? As a final lasting gesture before you motor away from the car park, you can't resist a look at your 'current' face, so you glance into your rearview mirror and quietly murmur at the face looking back at you – *'you are history, buddy, you unattractive, miserable, ugly git!'* Arriving home you pour yourself a glass of 'real orange juice' from the stale, half-full carton before keenly browsing through your new miracle purchase, and as promised on the cover by the author the 'life changing' tips begin to emerge: 'A daily walk is good for you, gets you into the fresh air where you'll get some 'free' Vitamin D'. You read on but already your eager, optimistic smile has been reduced to a grin, you're already a little disappointed but reassuringly you muse – this is just the foreplay, matey; you're convinced there is better to come! You turn the page quickly and more words of wisdom appear such as 'to avoid putting on weight try pushing the sugar bowl further away from your immediate grasp at the dining table, better still don't buy sugar during your weekly shop' and here's another tip: 'hide the salt cellar, you don't need it' and 'tighten your trouser belt up one notch, that's the idea' – cheap at the price, eh? Then you're informed: 'Swimming as an exercise is good for you, additionally it may prevent you drowning on your holiday in the summer sun!' Then there's a reassuring confirmation that 'strength training can be used to strengthen your body, and the following pages will show you how' and along come the press-ups! Now, for the first time since your costly purchase you begin to harbour doubts – but it's too late, buddy, you were too hasty in your purchase, you were conned, and there's no way the bookseller will contemplate a refund, and so, you are stuck with 'yet another 'miracle', quick fix H&F book (that's identical to the other 20 on your bookshelf), that's already on its way to Amazon to recoup a fraction of your expenditure.

In an attempt to bolster my struggling self-esteem, and in contrast to some other authors who release elaborate books on the health and fitness subject with no apparent credibility apart from their celebrity status, let me at this appropriate moment reassure you that I wouldn't willingly mislead you into any purchase of this book (in fact, I genuinely hope you've borrowed this one); I'm not interested in making money, honestly it's true; nor do I want to placate my well-earned anonymity all over the media. My reasons for writing are not at all based on business, I've started writing simply because I can and there's no reason why I shouldn't; also, currently I am bored rigid with little else to do at the moment other than partake in my usual quite mundane selfish daily activities, most of which still urge me to pull the sheets back at daylight before confronting yet another cold and bleak January morning. My views on life in general, but more so on health/fitness have been accrued over my current lifespan of 70 years, and although the views don't make me necessarily right, they are nevertheless different – not clever – but different as they are all based on the all-consuming lengthy 'athlete's' life I've led, and currently that's amounting to at least 66 plus years (and even before those 66 years when I was a tiny four year apprentice of physical 'activity'), as such, presumably it would be fair to say, there's at least a 'hint' of honest credibility!

Be kind to the elderly – many of us of a certain age come from a time when life was different, thoughts could be expressed and mocked without too much offence, work was social and practical jokes were looked forward to, a sense of humour didn't have to be analysed or approved, freedom of speech was second nature, and life was generally more diverse and therefore interesting.

I do feel uneasy though when offering negative comments aimed at other people, and with the above words I have at least hinted at some form of criticism, so before I continue let me just add, in terms of mentioning other authors, I have no real right (apart from Article 10 of the Human Rights Act which recognises our right to 'freedom of expression') to deal out a bit of negativity, nor do I have the right to really disapprove of other people's work – after all, who am I to compare and then criticise? However, on a personal basis, I honestly find it a bit depressing as well as unnecessarily egotistical to appear to criticise others, whilst conversely trying to create some credibility of my own. It would be much easier to praise, even if the subject is unpraiseworthy. However, I see my 'excuse' as being as much to do with the normal process of 'aging' which offers me some justifiable comfort on the basis that I've been around the block not once or twice but rather a few thousand times. Most of my sarcasm or cynicism, which grows annually, derives not from a bitter twisted person but rather from experiences gained over many years of involvement in life's arduous journey, and within that journey there's an inescapable accumulation of age-related negative baggage we all somehow accrue in our lifetime. With age, you see, as you'll discover soon enough, if indeed you aren't there already, there comes a shed load of baggage, that's baggage you inadvertently collect, store, and then cart around with each passing year of your life without even noticing its cumbersome presence, until perhaps you sit back in a moment of quiet solitude and somewhat belatedly you analyse your own views. In essence, and as horrible as it is, there is little new in life when you've reached a 'certain age', you've either 'seen *it before'*, *'heard it before'*, or indeed *'done it before!' – oh god what does that sound like?* And all that baggage quietly transforms you from the nice, always keenly excited, reasonable person you once were when younger into the unmistakable miserable old git you've somehow transcended into and which you truly never wanted to be or believed ever would be! But be honest, Mick, come-on now, you are, son, you're a miserable old git (who earnestly believes, every neighbourhood cat only ever shits on your veg patch), oh yes you are, you're a crest-fallen, poverty stricken, contemptible old weather-beaten crony, otherwise your nearest and dearest wouldn't keep telling you those home truths, now would they?

So, after a somewhat reflective pause to soak up the self-inflicted criticism, let's get back to this one-way discussion and in so doing return to some semblance of the intended subject! *I would state with a degree of sadness, that my presumed place as a very experienced practitioner within the subject of health and fitness now embarrasses me, and that's because I truly don't want to be associated within a section of society that has turned my once respected hands-on occupation, and all-consuming hobby, into a subject that appears to be designed 'for the lovely by the lovely' for the sole purpose of making money!* Although I hold the view that beauty is skin-deep, it seems currently that old, visually 'unpleasing', overweight people with spots growing out of spots and weather beaten wrinkled faces don't write books on health and fitness even if they have much to offer. Angels and Adonises fronting articles in newspapers, magazines or presenting the television shows are now both the custom and the norm.

What concerns me more than the trivia I've written above, is that today's subject authors and media, in all its varying forms, have turned a very 'simple subject' (health and fitness, for want of another term) into a perceived complicated difficult to understand science (part of which I hope to reverse), whilst at the same time the documentary presenters appear to be the vainest and most self-promoting prophets on the planet. My view is that general health and fitness is relatively simple, while illness and injury aren't. For many exponents it's a celebrity thing, the celebs have 'gotta get noticed' – somehow, or even anyhow, otherwise they'll not be celebs anymore, then what? They could even lose their eminence, god forbid, and become 'ordinary' arrrgh surely not! It seems there are currently just so many numerous youthful 'models', many of whom it seems are barely out of school, who pretend to want to 'inspire' other model types as they shine like a vision of beauty from the countless shiny magazine covers and state of the art gymnasiums. The books and articles they write are not intended for Mr and Mrs Ordinary. Most people presumably will look at the presentations and with a friendly smirk quickly realise it is all fantasy as they contemplate how they can integrate all that expensive and often elusive 'tosh' into their own busy lives, whilst continuing to work 40 hour weeks, feeding the kids, taking the dog out, attending school open days as well as doing the weekly supermarket shop, let alone book the car in for its MOT and annual service and cut the grass.

In contrast to the current assembly of youthful authors, many appearing barely out of their teens, 20 years ago I was 50 years old and about to begin another chapter of my sporting life, before going on to self-coach myself into winning at least (they're the result sheets I can find) 75 cycling races, that's between the ages of 50 and 61 (and at 61 I was riding 10 miles in 20m 25s). Before that I was again 'self-coached' and self-supported in winning the North Eastern Counties Marathon title, against 250 club 'athletes' from all over the country! Following that chaotic period as a decent club runner, I had 12 years as an amateur Triathlete winning 47 open events, and setting a new British Ironman record, whilst accumulating 18 British Championship medals along the way, as well as the wonderful honour of adorning a Great Britain tracksuit for almost a decade while working 40 hour weeks. Nearly forgot, before all of that I was a proud Royal Marine Commando for several energetic years representing the Corps in Boxing, Hockey, Athletics and Cross Country running, and finally, here I am leading up to today, and the last 10 years of my life (that's from 60 to 70) have been every bit as energetic, racing on a bike, setting records whilst finishing in the top three in Park Runs (and placing 11th from 557 finishers at 69 at another event); additionally I have recently had top 12 positions in Triathlons (from 250ish at 68 years of age) and even been 1st across the line in a Duathlon. Regardless of all the latter, I consider myself to be the most ordinary and unknown person on the planet. Now the latter sentence doesn't read right, but I figure you'll know what I mean. So somewhere within the globe of my self-confessed often redundant cranium there is a wealth of innate practical knowledge, the vast majority of which has been accrued through 'experience' as opposed to a course or two, or a book or two.

In concluding this early chapter, where I'm attempting to sell myself from the credibility perspective not dissimilar to how it works when attending a job interview, the one thing I am happy with is having 'lived the life' of an amateur athlete for decades, while remaining ordinary in everything else. Although it's not for me to say, I'll say it anyhow: my personal CV if closely analysed, especially in relation to credibility, should stand up well to 'intense scrutiny', and that's regardless of not being labelled as yet another professor, doctor or personal fitness trainer to the stars and celebrities, all of whom are apparently so well qualified to show the iconic famous people how to jog, touch their toes, and do bicep curls!

Occasionally as we work through the remaining pages of this amateur's book, I'll see if I can make any sense of it all before suggesting a different approach more befitting (no offence intended) *the ordinary, everyday person, that's you and I!*

To: *Dave Aylwin, John Hall, Ian Miller, Taff Bailey, George Storey, Dame Kirby and Robbo! Thanks for just being there and making me laugh, oh how I look forward to our next pint, lads, when we've kicked COVID into touch.*

You don't need endless repetitive studies and research projects to determine the general health and physical condition of a country's population! Just sit on a chair or a bench anywhere in a public domain, and simply *watch the world go by! OR – HAVE A QUICK LOOK AT HOW BUSY THE NHS IS? CURRENTLY IT'S NEVER BEEN SO LADEN!!!*

THERE IS A START, MIDDLE AND AN END TO EVERY THING

ON THAT BASIS – HOW'S OUR CURRENT HEALTH? 'WHERE ARE WE NOW IN THE YEAR 2021?' AND HOW HAVE WE ARRIVED AT THIS POINT?

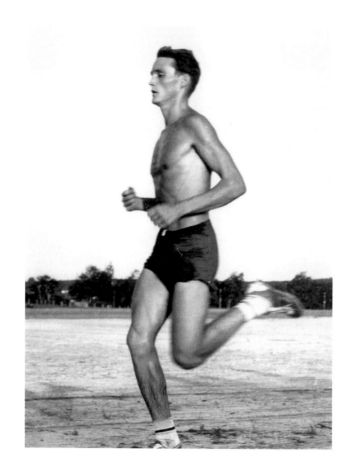

I've run all over the world, this is racing in the Far East, hence the lack of a vest.

MOVEMENT

*When you think about it, the existence and life of a human-being is made possible simply because of an action known as '**movement**', and when movement (kick-started and then governed by the heart) stops altogether, we die; therefore, movement is clearly fundamental to life itself. Isn't the latter blatantly obvious? Well, if that's the case, why then do the bulk of humanity stay so motionless for huge periods of their lives, not dissimilar to a motionless, camouflaged sniper hidden in the undergrowth? I'll stick my uneducated neck out and say movement in all its various forms is not just instinctively natural, it's also clearly an essential and crucial part of life itself! Most forms of movement are to a large degree based on instinct and with instinct we don't actually engage the brain, e.g. blinking, swallowing, scratching, stretching, sneezing, and even walking if only to the toilet. Try this: take a pencil or pen and run it very lightly over your lips, like a feather, or over your eyelashes – it's almost impossible not to 'respond', right? Well, that's a simple example of 'instinctive behaviour'. To fight the instinct* is to fight against life itself, to deny exercise is to fight instinct and is similar to being shot by 'friendly fire' – totally self-defeating, dead people don't move a lot either (so I'm told) which is just as well I guess (I've just shivered at the thought!). Yet vast portions of the human race, particularly within the Western world, or so it seems, would rather die unpleasantly and in quite major discomfort than move! During the lockdown over Covid, the government were encouraging us all to take exercise. Where I live, there are approximately 3,000 people (and we'll be no different from any other town or village in the UK), but only a 'tiny' percentage of us decided to exercise and at least take a 'walk', on the basis that it's healthy and good for us, as well as being declared by government as above board. Now during the Covid-virus, I could and indeed did walk every morning for 45 minutes, I did it for months with our dog and would barely pass a solitary soul – totally bizarre, eerie, in fact! Long streets empty, fields and footpaths deserted, woodland desolate apart from sparrows, blackbirds and the occasional robin. There are people close to where I* *live who I haven't seen once in months, I know they are alive simply because their bins go out once a week then somewhat mysteriously disappear later. Now it would appear the lockdown is coming to a fragile end, and of course we knew it would, but I wonder what effect the year of isolation and total inactivity will have had on so many people, as well as of course ultimately our National Health Service who at the end, pick up the bill. Some will, of course, say perhaps in a righteous way 'we were told to isolate' and that of course is true to a degree, but we were also told and 'encouraged' to take exercise and get outside if you are able; arguably it was easier to isolate 'outside' than in company indoors! YOU CAN LEAD A HORSE …! Again, I have occasionally witnessed people with a mask on, clearly observing the rules, but then at the same time sucking deeply on their killer cigarette every few seconds! Your point is?!! I'll interpret – the mask will keep me alive – but the cigarette will?!!! And Exercise? No chance. I might catch the 'virus'!*

*On the subject of instinct. In my occupational role with Northumbria Police, I was occasionally invited, or required, to attend a meeting designed to assess the actions of an on-duty police officer, perhaps following a complaint of 'unreasonable behaviour' or a 'use of force' issue, the actions having been caught on CCTV or even a bystander's mobile phone. Time and time again I'd see an officer respond to an incident which wasn't strictly in-line with training procedures, and the investigating officers often had people immediately found guilty simply because their actions weren't a carbon-copy of those in the official training manual, yet the training manual, which was a huge cumbersome publication, was never designed to be totally prescriptive, because there would always be incidents which were out of the ordinary or at least very unusual; in other words, there may have been occasions when an officer was unable to select an 'official' or recognised response option from the 'manual' because time was exceedingly short or the incident was itself rare and even bizarre and without precedent. I can remember footage of one such incident whereby an officer, having just arrived on the scene(as directed), had been immediately punched with excessive force squarely in the face by a drunk male. This occurred in a noisy public place, and within a 'split second' the officer responded with 'like', i.e. he punched the assailant back in the face! It was clear from where I was that the officer responded 'instinctively', in other words he had minimal time to make a considered training-related response; as such his reaction was hurried and fundamentally based on, amongst other things, a degree of fear, panic or even survival, brought on by the extreme nature of the assault in a noisy and hostile area (forget the uniform, police officers are first and foremost human-beings). From where I was, and clearly I wasn't an official Judge, his actions appeared proportionate, reasonable under the circumstances, and possibly even necessary, otherwise without a hasty response the assault on him may well have continued. Anyhow, you can see the link with another area associated with instinctive behaviour! *Interesting?* I was lucky in my work, a lot of it broadened my interest and knowledge on human behaviour, and in having a good imagination, ensured I could easily put myself in the place of another person certainly helped. Books can be absorbingly interesting, but reality is more compelling!

On a totally different issue, I would always tell my athletes to warm-up 'systematically' because it helps to be habit-forming; once again when athletic pre-event nerves and large amounts of adrenalin are flowing, working on habit-based actions can be beneficial, and limit or reduce elements of uncertainty. *Anyhow back to the subject!*

Guitar Slim once gleefully sang about his current poor health predicament – 'I've had my fun, if I never get well no more!' and I have to respect his sentiments; he was simply saying it was all my fault to be where I'm at I knew the risks as such I'll take the blame and the consequences. In contrast – how many of our country folk when seeking help from the NHS, will stand up and be counted due to their health issue being the result of a 'self-inflicted' illness? Then when treatment isn't immediately available will shout with venom at the inadequacies of the NHS!!

Here is something to consider, some actions are just so obviously self-defeating!

For many years now the common view, I think it fair to say, has been that anything apparently 'new' (or recently invented) which is designed and purposefully built to make our life 'easier' or physically more 'comfortable' for us, has to be celebrated and loudly applauded. How quickly some things change, often within the blink of an eye – for example, a newly invented 'product' quickly transfers from being a useful 'occasional' time and labour saving bonus, to becoming an absolute 'necessity' or an 'essential' everyday commodity that we can soon barely do without; in the process of change the new invention quickly renders another form of exercise redundant. As the 'new' product quickly takes hold, the 'old' manual activity slowly dwindles away whilst resigning itself to extinction and history. The arrival of the 'new product' which eradicates further the need to physically move, ensures that there's yet another partial decline in the man and woman's 'physical' status, as the physical action is eradicated from both 'brain and muscle memory' as yesterday's capacity to easily perform that once common physical task is quickly forgotten, and as such is speedily eradicated from both muscle memory and everyday life!

A place in the sun! Have you watched the programme? It seems 'everybody' wants a pool 'to look at' from the recliner, but nobody wants to swim in it, and if the intended property purchase entails a walk for groceries once or twice a week, well that just won't do either! How many 'able' people now get their weekly shopping delivered, rather than venture out, walk and carry! How many houses have lost their nature friendly and once attractive and easy to manage front lawn, to be replaced by yet another concrete parking space? Two days ago, I watched an advert on TV for a remote control to open and close your blinds!

Let's look again at the imagined, new and must have 'modern dream product' and its effect on modern lifestyles. And so as we expend even less energy (due to the brilliance of the new item), we predictably get fatter, and as we get fatter and more out of shape we somewhat predictably struggle to perform those once frequent and often so trivial and so elementary daily physical tasks. As our fitness declines, from a lack of movement, we 'somehow' subject ourselves to an array of health-related illnesses and self-inflicted diseases, such as heart disease! Learning to cope with the illness we've mysteriously developed leaves us miserable, and the misery goes hand-in-hand with a general feeling of unhappiness, and with the latter mood swings even begin to affect our nearest and dearest, that's those who are now referred to today by the modern day term known as our 'loved-ones'. Furthermore, as the developing health condition becomes gradually more serious, we seek the assistance of the disappearing and often elusive family doctor. We've moved on and things unfortunately get gradually worse, and predictably you now require some professional help and support and naturally you ring the clinic. Annoyingly, the phone at the clinic continues to ring, until at last the stressed-out receptionist finally says 'hello, Z Z Top speaking, how can I be of assistance?' Before the words are out of Z Z's mouth you subject her to an onslaught of verbal abuse with accompanying obscenities because they've had the audacity to inform you the sad and unavoidable truth 'there's a waiting list, I'm afraid and the earliest we can fit you in is February 2023, so sorry', in the meantime reassuringly Z Z adds 'you might want to try Boots or Superdrug'! Now the developing anticipated lengthening queue somewhat predictably ensures you become even more miserable and depressed, and the misery and depression leads you predictably to the now common 'contagious' tag of having 'mental health' issues, as you continue to pursue the assistance of the cash-strapped, limited services, and seemingly empty NHS!

AND ALL the above is perhaps indirectly derived from an unwillingness, or even an aversion, to *movement* and *exercise* and then to further complement the exercise try to eat a reasonably healthy and nutritious diet! HERE'S THE OH SO HATED TRUTH – 'IN LIFE AS WITH MOST THINGS – WE REAP WHAT WE SOW!' REMOVE PHYSICAL MOVEMENT FROM YOUR LIFE AND YOU WILL BECOME PHYSICALLY FEEBLE WITH MANY SELF-INFLICTED LIMITATIONS. EAT TOO MUCH FOOD AND GO NOWHERE EXCEPT THE CAR, THE OFFICE AND THE SITTING ROOM SOFA AND YOU'LL GET FAT, GET FATTER AND YOU WILL FURTHER ENCOURAGE OBSESITY, BECOME OBESE AND YOU'LL GET ILL, GET ILL AND YOU MAY DEVELOP MENTAL HEALTH PROBLEMS AS YOU INCREASINGLY BECOME DEPRESSED! Exercise is not a panacea, but ignore its importance in your daily life at your peril!

So, do yourself a huge unselfish favour, and in the process save a boat load of money. TAKE A WALK, EAT AN APPLE, SMILE and BREATHE DEEPLY (it doesn't have to be an embarrassing, eye-catching spectacle), then when no one's looking TRY A 10 METRE JOG, THEN WALK AGAIN until you've recovered, then try ANOTHER 10 METRE JOG before you WALK some more, and when no one's looking do a few ARM CIRCLES – your 'ball and socket' shoulder mechanism is specifically designed for that smooth circular motion (although it may have forgotten); after 20 minutes go and watch some television! Is it that simple? Yes, it's not too difficult – but more importantly it's a start!

Still on the same subject - have a quiet giggle (or a raucous side-splitting laugh) at the very clever universal boss! A *parody of the haves and the have nots! In the long run (excuse the pun), who wins?*

Most of my working life I have inadvertently discovered that people will go to great lengths to avoid anything that entails walking (getting your shopping delivered to your doorstep as mentioned above is one of those examples) and the *more important* you are judged to be, the less it seems you care to walk. Here's an example. When I worked at Northumbria Police Headquarters there was a constant everyday battle to find parking places, mainly due to an ongoing influx of weekly training courses etc. The ever-increasing amount of *'important'* people, that's those earning the most money, were deemed so valuable that they were given a special 'prize', their very own individual 'parking slot' that no one else was allowed into*. The eye catching, often empty, 2x3 metre bay even had its very own little sign carefully implanted on the hallowed site, in so doing identifying the importance of the bay's 'owner'. Furthermore, the special parking bays were situated as close as possible to the door of the 'VIP's' office, and there were loads of them, VIPs I mean. The rest of us (befitting our lowly, inexpensive positions) often had a daily yomp to our workplace from Car Park C as it was known, of 400 metres there in the morning and then 400 back in late afternoon. Now the latter, 'need to walk' was somehow seen as a level clearly befitting our less than important occupational status, or if you prefer, those of us earning much less money than those with a personal car-port. But as the saying goes, *there's a bunch of Daffodils in every dustbin and* here's the good news: the longer the walk from Car Park C to employee destination five days a week adds up to two and a half miles of exercise; not life changing perhaps but nevertheless…! BUT (I have just worked that out over the past three hours) and it comes to 120 miles a year of exercise!! And you didn't even notice it. The longer the walk, the healthier we became, the shorter the walk, well, the fatter and unhealthier we became – *and they thought they were bright!!!* I can't stop laughing – and even that's good for me! So arguably in their caring wisdom our 'superiors' were kindly ensuring that their employees lived a bit longer than themselves, even if it was with a bit less dough!

*On the subject of bosses and 'others', I was once sent down to London as a representative for Northumbria Police in a huge nationwide seminar at the Met. I was to travel with a good friend of mine called Dave Metcalfe, a Chief Inspector, but I was the force 'expert' in the subject material about to be discussed and debated. Even now, I'm still not really sure what Dave's perceived role was on this occasion (maybe there to see me through the underground safely?). Anyhow when we met at Newcastle's fine Victorian Station, we soon discovered Dave, because of his higher rank, had a First Class ticket, and me (on this occasion the 'expert') because of my 'lower' rank was to travel Second Class!! Anyhow, Dave being an ordinary decent bloke, and despite his obvious 'perceived' importance, sympathetically relented his First Class ticket and travelled in the second class compartment with his not so important lowly buddy who (someone, with a 'parking slot' no doubt had decided) was only good enough for a Second Class ticket. As we sped along down to King's Cross (out of respect, Dave had the window seat) as you'd expect, well, Dave read the huge broadsheet Daily Telegraph and I read the cheaper but easier to manage Sun. Anyhow, in line with the above chapter on the 'haves and have nots' of the workplace, well, I've 'decided' purely out of infantile spite, befitting a guy 'without a car parking space', that I'll out-live Dave by a decade or two and go to his funeral rather than him come to mine!! Because, similar to the above, on arriving home to the Toon, well, Dave opted for a taxi, and me? Well, I 'walked' up to the Haymarket, and used up another three calories, which wasn't much but it was three more than him!! *Dave, by the way, was a fit guy and always had the common sense to work out regularly!*

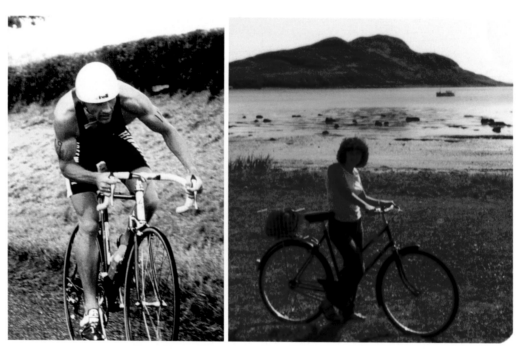

Recreation or racing, either way they both burn fuel (calories) and both exercise the engine (Cardio). There are many health promoting options to choose from.

Habit

(the invisible scourge)

THE BEGINNING OF A HABIT IS LIKE AN INVISIBLE THREAD, BUT EVERY TIME WE REPEAT THE ACT WE STRENGTHEN THE STRAND. ADD TO IT ANOTHER FILAMENT UNTIL IT BECOMES A GREAT CABLE AND BINDS US IRREVOCABLY, THOUGHT AND ACT. (Orison Swett Marden)

(I wrote the following small article 21 years ago
for a work-related book I authored)

Every day I am privy to people who, by virtue of habit, wake up, walk 10 metres to their car, arrive at work and park at the nearest accessible point to their office, sit down for an average of seven hours, then reverse the pattern homeward. At college, I see the vast majority of people queue instinctively for as long as it takes to use the lift rather than save time and walk two or three flights of stairs. At weekends, I see neighbours who take the car from the garage and actually drive 200 metres for the Sunday papers, rather than walk, and at Christmas (at the time of writing it's topical) I see offspring hypnotised by computer, phone, television and video. No longer do bikes, skates, and games of twenty-a-side traditionally clog up the streets.

Then I see people, miserable and dissatisfied with their physical condition and appearance.

Well you know, as I've said a million times, 'you reap what you sow'!

Presumably you are where you are because, that's where you want to be. If you want to be somewhere else – move (pun intended)! You want to be fit and healthy? Easy – work at it just a bit. You get nothing for nothing, if it's worth having, it's worth working for – try as hard as you like, but passing the buck onto the National Health Service is a poor and selfish choice!

As mentioned, I wrote the above article for a workbook I authored in 2000. Have we got healthier since that self-penned factual expression? Ha, I think not! Someone wrote lately, and not for the first time – we Brits are the fat man (and woman) of Europe. I wonder why?

The good news is, of course, obvious, and that is: it doesn't have to be that way. So let's not be too negative and accept that for most of us we can begin another of life's chapters by looking forward with optimism to improved health, it's a sound philosophy, and one I used to include those days when I did regular pre-retirement talks. Those days as part of my introductions my opening line was *'shortly you'll all have the opportunity to be a lot healthier and fitter than you've been for the past 40 years'! Because the future is still yours and mine to mould, AREN'T YOU LUCKY?* Listen, even Noddy Holder bellowed with optimism in his celebrated Christmas song 'look to the future now it's only just be g u u un'! In so doing I assume Noddy was hinting that the old was somehow lacking and the new had much better prospects.

Of course, what has been is now gone, and only history books and our mind with its countless stored memories can bring it temporarily back. Although we can reflect on things gone, we clearly can't change the past; apart from perhaps obliterate it by distasteful brutish actions such as using extreme force to drag a 200-year statue, which has stood the severe test of time, down from its plinth before dumping it into several feet of murky water! Get a life!! Anyhow, that's another matter, regardless of our somewhat ferocious and compulsory appetite to replace old with new, I'd suggest that there is an emergence of available information compelling us (if we can only but see it) to compare the past with the current and in so doing invite us to contemplate a 'partial' return to aspects of general living in simpler times; I am clearly suggesting there was real credence with some stuff that was once the norm in the past.

Looking at issues within the world now in 2021, most of which affect the ordinary working class citizen, there is a lot to contemplate about the current way of living; in fact, there's times when it appears the whole world is falling apart at the seams and similar to an encroaching massive tsunami which rapidly engulfs everything within its mighty path there's little it seems that we can do to prevent the slide. In my autobiography I wrote about growing up through the post-war years of the 1950s and the colossal change that occurred in society within those times and then into the wonderment of the 1960s and 1970s. Writing a separate lengthy book about those years, how we thought and how we lived etc would not be difficult as there was so much new happening then, and those years provided happy memories for many of us; interestingly, **where were issues about mental health then?** But, here's a question that sits comfortably within the broad spectrum of this book; the question, I have to admit is not straightforward but it conveniently takes me into another chapter even if the question is difficult to answer, nevertheless here it is. 'Although arguably we had much less in years gone by in terms of commodities, *'were we, the people, wealthier, happier and indeed 'healthier' during the 1950s and into the 1960s than we are today in 2021, and that's regardless of all the modernisation and advances made in the past few decades?'* Well I was there then, and clearly I'm still here now, so let's go back and have a look!

A famous general apparently once said 'we aren't retreating; we are simply advancing in a different direction'.

Note: Although the above notes are linked to a lot of the chapters which follow, here's a final sentiment for consideration on the demise of health in 2021 Great Britain!

Straight from a Queen song – where is the next one coming from? All the following professional occupational titles have recently (within a two-week spell) been taken from articles in newspapers, supplements, and television programmes advising on how to improve health, whilst in the process acquiring a physically fit body, just like the presenters. A regular occurrence during the programmes is the following: While the trim, well-manicured, youthful presenter has a well-earned rest she/he is replaced by 'another professional', whose job specific title comes straight out of the almanac of 'Obscure and never heard of Professions', and the intro goes along the lines of *'So to find out more, I went to see '...' a ... to seek their professional advice'*! It seems there's an endless list of experts* as such, take your pick from the selection below! **Here for your perusal are the following! Which one of those specified below do you need?**

* Before that, though, a question: **When do an array of practitioners turn a corner and join the hallowed ranks of people now referred to as 'experts' and *who* promotes the pro from just another person doing their job, with an additional title who's now all of a sudden referred to as an 'expert'!** I mean we see people who one minute are presenting practical fitness sessions and the next authoring books on Healthy Eating with a boat load of graphic, mouth-watering recipes. Wonder what 'proper' chefs think about that? And how 'proper' fitness exponents would feel about Chefs writing fitness books while jumping energetically around sitting rooms? Anyhow!

Professors (there's millions of them – what do they do when not on the telly?), Doctors 'of' etc. (many thousands, but few it seems in the clinic), Scientists (yip there's countless) – <u>anybody know a plumber?</u> – Physiotherapists, Biologists, Associate Professors of Exercise, Practitioners of Clinical Endocrinology and Metabolism, Exercise Physiologists and Members of England Panel, Professors of Medicine and Metabolism, Pharmacists, Brain Fitness Experts, and Body Coaches as well as 'A' doctor who is the Clinical Lead for Headache Service, there's Nutritional Therapists, a Doctor Consultant in Anaesthesia, and Wellness Practitioners, Psychosexual Therapist, also we've got Yoga experts and 'A' Noted Dietitian, there's Professors of Experimental Psychology – <u>anybody seen an electrician?</u> – Chiropractors, 'A' Doctor who's a Consultant in Dermatology. There's a 'top' Neurologist (are there any 'bottom' ones?), and there's a Psychotherapist and Mental Health Consultant. Social Prescribers of Well-Being are kicking about, and today for the first time there's a new kid on the block referred to as a Breath Work Coach (where have you come from?)! Oh, hang on, there's also Mental Health Activists and Brain Fog exponents and a Pet Bereavement Coach, Menopause Coach, a Divorce Coach, a Retirement Coach and a Dating Coach. Finally, last but by no means least, there's the much sought-after god-like Personal Fitness Trainers to the 'Stars' and 'Celebrities'! We've also got a boat load of modern day well-equipped Gymnasiums opening (and unfortunately just as quickly closing), and 'Uncle Tom Cobley and all', they're all just like the model presenter to help us get fit! At a price, of course. Think I'll just take a walk and eat an apple or two.

Wait a minute now I'm still here, and I'm not quite finished – additionally, or so it seems, there are just thousands of 'Personal Fitness Trainers' going way back to Cilla's Saturday night Blind Date show and must see television programme which opened along the following lines: – 'Who are you, number 3 and where do you come from?' –*'Hi Cilla, my name's Anthony, I'm nearly 17 and a Personal Fitness Trainer from Grimsby'* (names are fictional) or *'Hi Cilla my name's Henry, I'm 16 and a half and I'm also a Personal Fitness Trainer from the Shetlands, and rowing and hill climbing are my specialist subjects'!*

Despite all the above (and the list grows even as I write,) and all their books, on-line sitting room work-outs, videos and telly programmes, together with page after page of their succulent Mediterranean recipes (with a 'gram' here and a 'calorie' there), all designed to 'inspire' and educate us all in a revolution in healthy living.

After all that – and all those teams of 'health and fitness experts', well, would you believe it, the nation's health and physical fitness mysteriously 'declines' and has quite possibly never been worse, as the ambiguous additional subject of Mental Health issues joins us and apparently accelerates quicker than bog rolls leave the shelves during Covid!

To Ossie, Ronnie, Alan, Cease, Willie, Keith, The Bant, Ivan, Henna and Alec! 65 plus years – memories! Am I lucky or am I lucky!

To Mary, Irene, Lynn, Christine, Susan, Carol, Judith, Karen, Julie and Christine. Martyrs that's what you are – and you even sleep with them! So brave!

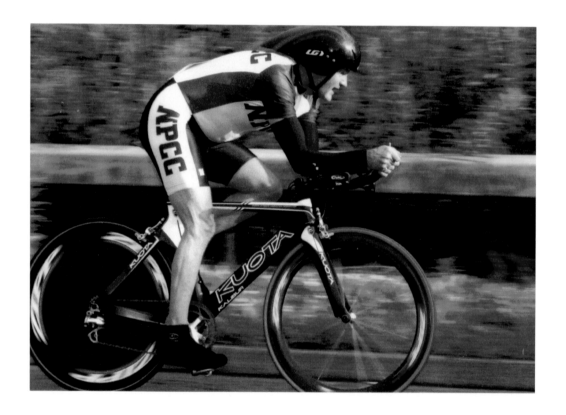

To Tim Miley, my team racing partner, and thanks
for keeping your 'admin' eye on me! All the best.

ONCE UPON A TIME!

Keeping in line with the title of this book, especially the '70 year' term I've used – let's go back a while, close to my beginning, for in total contrast to the ever-growing list of health, fitness, wellness, mental health and Brain experts and the prolific opening of Sport Centre gymnasiums and personal home gymnasiums that are in abundance in 2021, well, in total contrast, in 1956 rural Northumberland there wasn't even a clinic – as a babe I was pushed in a pram to the lounge of the local Working Man's Club for nurses' inspections (possibly where I discovered a liking for beer?). IN CONTRAST, WHAT WE HAD WAS 'A' DOCTOR AND 'A' MULTI TASKED SINGLE TEACHER DEPLOYED TO A CLASS OF 40 CHILDREN TO TEACH 'EVERYTHING' INCLUDING MATHS, ENGLISH, RELIGIOUS EDUCATION, GEOGRAPHY, HISTORY, NATURE STUDIES AND EVEN 'PHYSICAL EDUCATION'! HERE'S HOW IT WORKED!

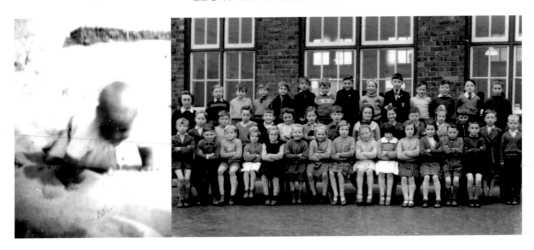

"On your marks, get set!"
Me in 1951...

...and again in 1957. I'm seated third from left with my school buddies, there's not a picking on any of us and mental health wasn't even invented.

Doctor Danny O'Driscoll* speaks quietly in a beautiful soft Irish accent as he welcomes a local member of the community into his small study! *'Hello Margaret,' he begins with a half-smile, 'lovely to see you, take a seat please.'* The much respected doctor's local knowledge is immediately evident – *'how's your father?', 'and your mother Margaret, how is she?', 'and Mary, is she well?', followed by a gentle nod before, 'and Robert, a soldier now I hear?', 'how's Linda, she'll be six now?' 'And how's young Michael, still running around, I trust?', 'and you, are well, Margaret?'* he finally enquires with a nod!

Once upon a time, 65 years ago, in the small Northumbrian village of Widdrington, there was a doctor's surgery which took place in a small room within the doctor's own house; internal furniture and specialist 'tools of the trade' consisted of a small portable heater, two chairs, a stethoscope and an assortment of bandages and Elastoplasts, as well as some medicinal products, all of which will be administered by the much respected and well-liked doctor.

Half a mile through the adjacent well-trodden woods there was the red brick community school, which stood within 100 metres of the local Colliery (the 'pit'). Within the school there were several classrooms and within each classroom there was one form teacher responsible for the assorted education of approximately 40 pupils. Even now, some 60 plus years later, it's not difficult to view several run-of-the-mill 1930s, 1940s or 1950s class school photographs, which act as a visual reminder and even a historical portrait, whilst also enabling a viewing of 40 intrigued, smiling pupils. The photos were taken adjacent to an old red brick school classroom, some children stood on wooden forms, the lucky ones sat on them, and picked up a spelk or two in their bums, and others at the front kneeled on 'coconut matting'. The photograph I'm looking at currently, displays all the various local children, both boys and girls all mingled together, wearing an array of interesting 'hand-me-down' clothing – the transfer of the clothing was normal by the way and wouldn't be referred to with the inclusion of the word 'poverty' attached to it, as perhaps it would be today. It is no secret to reveal that all the would-be 'models' that day appear slim or perhaps even thin (I feel a song coming on) and maybe some like me were also, and without wanting to appear unkind, slightly dim; regardless, all the kids were undeniably *fit and healthy;* additionally, none of those present had developed 'mental health' issues, and that's probably because the term 'mental health' was as rare as a shilling (5p) in the pocket of a child. In 1956 the kids had never heard or come across the term, so presumably it's fair to suggest therefore that mental health issues didn't really exist! Now 65 years later, there's a mental health 'epidemic', everybody's gone loopy, or so it seems – it's contagious, you see, and the method of spread is by virtue of a continuous, never ending reference to the term as well as numerous presentations and mental health conversations, so much so, that just like a covert mystical disease, you analyse it and the more you analyse it the more likely it is that you've now picked it up as well, arrrgh help!! The rise, it seems, is unavoidable, it's almost fashionable. I mean the celebs and royalty as well as sporting stars all have it! Just yesterday I saw a 'nine year old' boy giving a television interview (as they do) on his 'anxiety attacks'. Nine years old – where the hell has he picked that term up from? Shouldn't he be playing football, practising his 'keepy-ups' or cooking cakes, playing cowboys and Indians or gathering conkers (with his hard-shell helmet and safety goggles on – of course!).

I was one of those 40 class members (I can still real off all the names of my 40 classroom childhood buddies) and all of us in those four ranks had very similar lives. For example, we all lived in rented properties, council, colliery, or farm and as central heating hadn't reached us yet, coal fires were the 'fashion', additionally with few cars clogging up the streets we all had no option but to walk or 'even' run everywhere (can you imagine? Bah 'hard times', was it BB King who sang that?). As there was no Health and Safety then, so, few physical restrictions were imposed on the kids, nothing it seemed intruded on our young lives and so with a degree of instinct we did what came naturally, we walked, ran, skipped, climbed, shared the journey on a friend's bike whilst sitting comfortably on the cross-bar, jumped and even (I feel another song coming on) thumped each other.

Those days, for breakfast (sounds Dickensian I know) I had bread and jam, or occasionally dripping and bread; for myself and Linda (my older and much wiser sister), the bread and jam became surplus to current requirements, that's because waking up hungry is unusual – many of us eat breakfast because it is expected of us, although put cereal that has a sugar or chocolate coating in front of kids and you can be sure they will eat it. For Linda and me though, once our mother had left the kitchen I can clearly remember us biting the middle portion out of the sandwich before throwing the remaining crusts out of sight beneath a curtain which hid unsightly pots and pans under the kitchen sink. Once suitably fed and watered, my daily journey as a five year old was a **mile in length** (as the 'crow flies') and you can still tread that well-worn path from 79 East Acres to Stobswood School, with a vigorous nod from my handsome head whilst looking back. I'd say this journey was considerably further than that measured mile, as I'd zig zag along while shouting at the company of friends as I went. So, this infant in short pants would leave the house in all weathers with Linda shortly after 8am for a school start time of 9.00am, no parental guidance necessary. As mentioned, I wore short pants and Linda a skirt – kilts seemed to be a girl's fashion item then as I recall. My first pair of slightly big 'tough boys shoes' as they were advertised, were second hand 'hob nailed' boots (handed down to me from my cousin John) with the toes stuffed with newspaper to make them 'fit properly!'. When it rained or when there was snow on the ground, we wore wellies which rubbed endlessly on gastrocnemius and soleus muscles (see, I am indeed an expert!) – the latter is our bared 'calves' – causing unsightly red rims on our young developing lower leg muscles. At school, before being allowed into classrooms, our hands were roughly examined for dirt, on the basis that they had often accumulated muck from the woods, so we hastily spat on them to remove the 'germs' or worse they were hastily scrubbed in the freezing toilet tap water, before being hastily dried on our family knitted woollen jumpers. In 2021, and somewhat differently to 1956, this week as the kids returned to school after the enforced lockdown they are greeted with loving smiles, cuddles, accompanied by loud clapping applause by all the wonderful teaching staff!

TO: Mrs *Gagie (standard 2) I hereby forgive you, Miss, and your use of my increasingly red arse as the daily punch bag! In the words of my mother: 'well, Michael, she'll not have battered you for nothing, son!'*

Before lessons commenced we had the obligatory assembly where we heartily sang Christian hymns ('to be a pilgrim' or maybe 'for those in peril on the sea' or the engaging, easy to understand 'all things bright and beautiful'). We then pressed together our saliva-soaked gooey hands and prayed. Looking back at my childhood Christian upbringing, it seemed essentially that for children everything was eminently simple and easy to understand, the message was simple: 'be kind, treat all living things with respect and you may go to heaven'. Apart from our catchy rhythmic hymns, where the worded content was easily understood, we also prayed for a life that wasn't selfish (that's apart from reaping the wonders of heaven if we behaved ourselves, helped all other living things), and if we went off the straight and narrow (and got caught) we'd be caned, then we were advised to pray for forgiveness and move on. The hymn 'All things bright and beautiful' just about sums up our childhood vision and undoubted beauty of the world, and was one of those cheerful, ever optimistic Christian hymns, that just oozed the wonders of God's world. After all of that, we went to our respective classrooms. At approximately 10.30 we had a **20-30 minute exercise break** (known appropriately as 'play time') and a 'compulsory' free bottle of milk each, the milk was gobbled down in double quick time and the remainder of play time was eagerly spent running around the yard playing an assortment of energetic games; the weather was never a barrier. Back to class 20-30 minutes later (entailing a possible PE lesson! In the clothes and footwear we attended school in) till 12.00 or thereabouts and it was dinner time. Our food was what I'd call a replica of a coal miner's bait – there was no menu, you sat down and ate what was placed in front of you. The only real option as I remember was the tetties (potatoes) where there was a choice: you could opt for either one scoop or two, three or four! Accompanying the tetties (we never got chips or anything fried) were meatballs, mince, liver or fish etc, plus cabbage (the latter seemed obligatory as I remember) and carrots, peas and gravy, followed by a 'pudding' of rice, tapioca, apple crumble and custard etc, all freshly cooked in the adjoining kitchen by local women, no doubt supplementing their husbands' meagre 'pit wages', and all washed down with tap water to drink, end of! Back to the yard for a hastily arranged **game of 20-a-side football** before the bell summoned us back into class. Another break (play time) at two o'clock for **20-30 minutes of frenetic energy-sapping run arounds,** back to class for about 90 minutes before a final song – the first line going 'now the day is over, night begins to fall, shadows of the evening pass across the sky?' and that acted as the finale to end the day's 'studies'. **The one mile home run began at 3.30pm.** Once home my 'good hob nailed boots' were quickly replaced with the remnants of an old worn out pair of 'tough boys shoes', a sugar and bread sandwich or two was hastily eaten before being washed down with a cup of tap water and out we went back into the streets for an array of self-made physical games. In for dinner, a glance at the tiny black and white television screen before being commanded 'bed'! **Once under the covers our small infantile bodies wallowed in a deep sleep till 'reveille' and so to another day of scran, exercise, studies, exercise, studies, scran, exercise, studies, exercise, sugar 'n' bread, exercise, dinner and oh no, not bed time!!!**

With few cars available to offer lifts, most of the population used the services of 'United bus Service'. To take up your position in the friendly queue at a bus stop, you had at least a half-mile walk; once at the shopping destination, in the absence of supermarkets, you trailed up and down the respective high streets before queuing again for the journey home again and a half-mile walk home with all the bags for company.

About 20 years ago, I remember my mother looking casually out of the sitting room window before enquiring, *'Michael, what's happened to all the young lasses?'* – *'How'd you mean, Mam?'* I replied. *'Why are they all so 'big', son? We weren't like that when we were pushing prams and pushchairs – were we?'* Before rounding off with: *'there wasn't a picking on any of us, can you remember?'* By the way, my mother wasn't trying to be in any way offensive (she loved everybody!), it was purely an observation!

And so, and in summary, in 1956 there were 40 children in my first 'infants' class, we were all thin, or maybe slim, with some maybe even replicating me – thin as well as maybe just a bit dim!

And getting back on track, because this is meant to be a book labelled a 'seventy-year experiment in health and physical training' beginning around 1955, and it's 2021 as I write. I am 70 years old now and still running a two-mile time trial at six minute mile pace, cycling under the hour for 25 miles, swimming in lakes comfortably for up to an hour, whilst combining those activities into Triathlon competitions and finishing in the top 12, running Park Runs and almost always in the top 10 from 'hundreds' (even as high as 2nd) whilst in the process setting records, and in my 'spare time' walking the dog and converting a building site into a highly productive allotment! And yesterday morning at 7.30am on the 23/5/2021 I finished 5th 'overall' in a Duathlon, despite being in the 70 year-old category. The event comprised a 2.65km run, 20km cycle, and culminating in a 5.75run. So come on now, Doctor, tell me – I got it all so very wrong!

Despite the latter, if I die tomorrow, well, at least I'll die fit!

And so, what you have above is a brief summary of my daily life from five years of age, up to 11 years of age, beginning in September 1956 and commencement of my schooling. Those few years before school it appears that I simply annoyed everyone by getting in the way, as my dad once said, 'an energetic flaming nuisance' followed everywhere by the manta *'someone grab him for a minute'* to around sometime in 1962 at which time I was ordered to another school (no, not a 'bad lads' school, Ossie –cheeky git!); this time, however, we became civilised as such, we were 'transported' there in a school bus, and now attired for the first time in a smart uniform (trying desperately hard to learn how to tie a tie)which wouldn't gather muck from the journey, but due to our developing adult status we'd now probably begin to gather fat instead of muck, as our daily habitual exercise was substantially reduced.

To Mr Harry Clark (Stobswood School's Headmaster). *In 1958 I received a truly abysmal end of term school report – still got it, yet despite all those large numbers of kids under your charge, you somehow (from where?) realised I could perhaps offer something else apart from academics, as you commented that 'Michael has other qualities – other than academic!' Your comment assisted maybe because I was 'backstop' in the school's rounders team, or inside right in football. Oh how I would love to climb those stairs again (not this time for the cane though) up to your* *office with its coal fire and dusty hearth, place my books down on your desk with the inkwell, smile and say 'for you, boss, thank you for your faith!' RIP.*

In contrast to 1956! Straight off the press in February 2021 – A headline reads – the UK is 'fat man' (and woman 'presumably') of Europe, obesity, diabetes and heart disease are all on the increase as over 1,000,000 people are admitted to hospital because of obesity related illness, whilst one in every three children and two in every three adults are over-weight (somewhat contradictory, poverty is on the increase). There are some 7.6 million people who suffer from heart disease and five million have diabetes. Watch those stats increase very soon because thousands have 'willingly' locked themselves away whist sheltering in houses from the virus, and that's regardless of being regularly *encouraged* by the government to get out and 'exercise' daily.

I must point out that at no time in writing this book have I gone looking for statistics, all those numbers I have included above have appeared either on the television, radio and in newspapers. And now the pandemic is seemingly under control, the main everyday topic is back to 'eating out', socialising in pubs and 'holidays in the sun' with people apparently desperate to have the holidays 'they deserve' after lockdown kept us all inside!

And so, being born in 1951 and pre-school from the age of one year to three years it appears that I simply annoyed everyone by getting in the way – 'an energetic flaming nuisance' my dad called me, and being followed everywhere by the mantra of 'grab him for a minute'! After writing this (and you reading it), I'll still be annoying people!

Following on from this:

LET'S TALK EXERCISE

(an exhilarating gift or a cumbersome chore)!

Our (that's yours and mine) 'current' standard of personal fitness is like confetti at a wedding, here today but whisked away by the wind tomorrow. If you don't keep working at it, it will evaporate and melt into oblivion like a saucer of milk in the sun!

With all things health-related, 'longevity' should be the supreme aim, so don't stop!

To define the word exercise, I've cheated and just had a quick glimpse through my Collins Little Gem English Dictionary (yes, they're still in circulation although mine is 'obviously' well worn) and *exercise* is defined in short as *'the use of limbs for health'* and of course that's partially correct but there is so much more to it than that, so as such we need to expand on the term. I'd describe the latter portrayal as a quaint, rather meek view, undermining the importance of the word 'exercise' and its immensely important place within all our lives. As mentioned, the brief abridged description is by no means wrong, but the magnitude of exercise in terms of its importance within the subject of health is monumental, its importance is surpassed (in my opinion) only by the subject of nutrition (and I'll come to that soon). What is obvious is that all moving parts, that's those bits and pieces designed to move, should be engaged in movement at regular intervals – to leave them static and unemployed is to label them as redundant and therefore resign them to history. From toes and fingers, head and neck, shoulders and arms, chest and back, and of course lower limbs, there is an inherent need to keep them healthy, and we keep them healthy by moving them the way they were intended. Be careful with movement though – body parts are designed to move within certain limits, some rotate (circles), whist others move laterally, some bend and others stretch; anyhow move them in a fashion which is contrary to their design and there is a real risk of injury, by and large pain is the warning sign and not to be ignored. Here's an example of moving a body part outside of its normal range and the potential repercussions of doing so. In the police force of old, a certain amount of restraints were 'officially' used by operational police officers (and were medically validated), as types of controlling techniques, i.e. perhaps used to control an angry, non-compliant, dangerous person, the restraint or escorting techniques were partially successful because of the discomfort they placed on the detainee, and pain can be quite a major de-motivator. The words 'pain compliance' are no longer used and are seen today as not applicable, that's because the term caused a certain amount of anxiety and concern within the Legal fraternity, suggesting that a degree of torture was being used to control an individual, as such possibly may even be an infringement of Human Rights. The example I've used regarding moving something against its natural range is similar in theory at least to taking a limb or similar to a place where it struggles to go, and despite the obvious warning signs, if we persist, by trying to 'force' it there, an injury could well be the ultimate result. Picking up the thread again, ultimately the more regularly you move, the more supple you will be (as long as you adhere to a bit of common sense re its range) – simple as it sounds, keep the body well-oiled (synovial fluid secretes some moving parts by commencing movement) and the greater will be its efficiency. See chapter on mobility/flexibility.

The human body is so incredibly complex, contemplating its workings for as little as five minutes could turn you into a religious fanatic, as you ponder where and how it was all made. This absolute miracle of ingenuity that is the human form, can run 100 metres in 9.2 seconds or cover 26 miles in under two hours, its intelligence can be used to put people on the moon, its physical capacity can guide a ball, a little bigger than a kid's marble into a tiny hole in one swipe, at 600 metres, using what amounts to as a stick to strike it, we can also make clones of ourselves (free) whilst laughing hysterically at the absolute joy of it all. What's almost more implausible, considering all the intricacies of the human body, is that the maintenance of it is relatively simple. And isn't that just wonderful? Additionally, if you are reasonably fit and as yet free from medical issues, you can manage the maintenance yourself, you truly don't have to pay for 'professional' help, as you would if your car broke down or your laptop malfunctioned. For simple body maintenance, trust me, you don't have to pay as some within the fitness industry would have you believe.

Having read the above explanation, do something you rarely or perhaps never do: sit back for a minute or two and contemplate this idiot's statement whilst at the same time, consciously test the body's ability to automatically function in so many various ways. Go on, do it, blink your eyes, scratch your temple, wiggle your toes, make a fist, swallow, change your facial expression, nod, rotate your shoulders, write your name, send a message, smile and grimace ... Now additionally, try this, if you have children and grandchildren smile and have a look at them, if they aren't with you in person close your eyes – and look for them anyhow, do it without going anywhere or even leaving your seat, we carry them with us always, in our mind's-eye and can meet by simply thinking of them! Without getting weird, tune into your body, which means simply think about it, marvel at it like we do a newborn child. Maintenance of thousands of humanistic actions and having it work well derives from feeding it fuel and liquid – the best you can afford... Additionally nourish this marvel with an occasional pint of Guinness and a bag of 'Cheese 'n' Onion'! Servicing the body's 'movable parts' is just as easy, although a little more time consuming. At the risk of repetition, I'll say it again: it's not difficult to kickstart your body into an agreeable, tailor-made for you, physical activity.

The *improvement* and *maintenance* of general health will be sadly lacking a major ingredient if we don't consider the use of EXERCISE in all its various and numerous forms, as part of the overall programme. The body was never designed to stay still for long periods, apart from some well-earned rest and recuperation following activity.

TWO words are ever relevant and present in exercise, the words apply regardless of whether you are a world-leading athlete or like the vast majority of us an ordinary run of the mill geezer – the words? **DISCIPLINE AND CONSISTENCY! Reality is harsh, though, and the reality is that 'no-one can do your exercise for you', and that's why 'discipline' is such a vital key, marry that up with 'consistency' and you can see the link.**

What type of exercise is best? There's not an immediate or precise answer to that, and that's because as individuals we are all so very different. When I worked at my last job with thousands of personnel to cater for, I regularly received phone calls requesting what would appear on the whole to be a pretty simple request. Typically: *"Mike, dee us a favour, man, me missus says am ower fat and if a keep gannin al borst, ind she doesn't want to redecorate afor Christmas, send us a training programme, man, so's al get some peace!"* It pays to remember the obvious; as mentioned, **we are all so very different.** Take two Olympic athletes in the same event, both at the pinnacle of physical perfection, yet both in that position by virtue of totally differing methods of preparation. Try not to copy, it's daft; what suits one may be a disaster and totally inappropriate for another. Considerations including aim, gender, size, physique, past history, available time, ability, current state, likes and dis-likes and availability of facilities, strengths and weaknesses, should all play a role in the individual training programme. On countless occasions I've been privy to groups of people with purple complexions covered in sweat, with protruding eyes and teeth marks on bottom lips, egging each other on to complete 5 reps of an outlandishly excessive weight when one rep is probably too much for at least three-quarters of the group. Apart from male machismo, misdirected competitive spirit and short lived satisfaction, WHAT IS THE POINT? And furthermore, how long in terms of weeks, months or years is it all likely to continue for? Unless it's for competitive purposes where the 'overload' principle is a crucial factor in improvement, what you do today should be repeatable and possible tomorrow and in the years ahead; *consistency* is so very important – you often lose fitness quicker than the time it takes to gain it. Television adverts are often 'incredibly misleading', they suggest, by use of the slim-line models, that high intensity workouts are the holy grail. Now, there is a place for 'harder efforts', but I'll tell you over and over again (for the non-competitive athlete) 'pain is a big de-motivator' – if it always hurts like hell – one day 'soon' you'll get out of your cosy warm little bed and say "Aye … that, not today!" What a waste!! Look for a balance in your efforts – easy, harder, easier, steady, harder, and even a 'good fun relaxed' ingredient. See chapter on 'Cross Training' and learn the principles, of how to safely improve or maintain your desired levels of fitness, dream a little if you must, but above all be a realist. As mentioned before, you are unique, you are special!

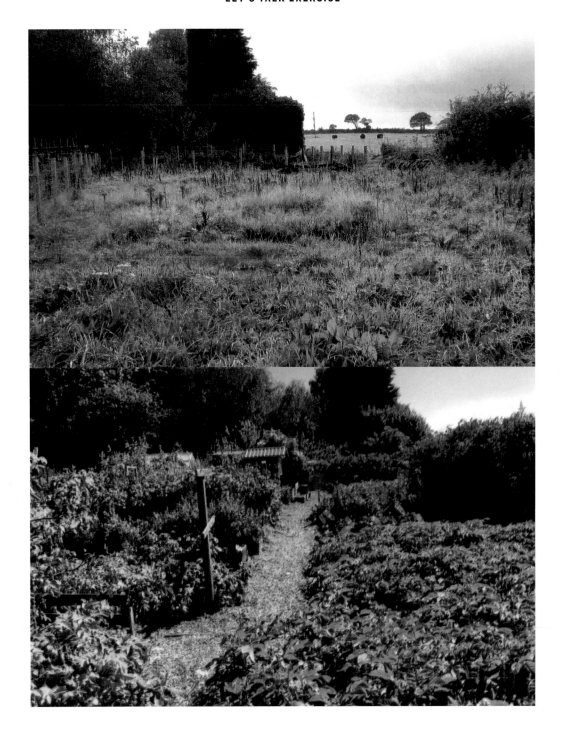

It took me several weeks to change a building site into a highly productive allotment, different exercise perhaps, but all good.

There are numerous forms of exercise on the menu, from digging your allotment to sprinting up a steep hill, to taking the stairs three at a time, and you choose from the menu what suits you personally, after reflecting on your personal aims and what you want to achieve, as well as the all-important personal issues such as time availability and what you are currently physically capable of. We'll look at various possible exercise assortments soon. Here's a *cautionary* note, though. Before they banned smoking adverts there was always a health-orientated warning that went with the product, i.e. in bold lettering on the actual carton, and that warning went with the eye-catching *smoking kills logo*. Yet currently and somewhat conversely, the 'vast' majority of fitness linked **adverts** and presentations on the television have few such health warnings, and these adverts don't show what I'd call the 'ordinary' person; rather, they show 'young' made to look like 'athletic models' (male and female) performing 'frenetic' exercise routines, and by frenetic I mean 'flat out' –'don't you dare stop me', gut busting, exhausting workouts – mostly performed on a trendy expensive fitness item such as a brand new and previously unused static exercise bike or something similar. The absolute joy the 'athletes' exhibit (remember they are getting paid to look this happy) both during and on conclusion of the ride or exercise, or so it seems, is very close to orgasmic with eyes rolling skyward as they alight from the bike and slither and slide across a room on the sweat covered floor, smiling as if sipping a pint of ice-cold Guinness, as they speedily make their way to a fridge full of colourful health drinks, ugh, probably accompanied by bonny coloured pills and an assortment of other miracle, heaven-sent supplements. The sweat-soaked Adonis is now laughing like a heaven-sent sporting Angel. All designed, of course, to have us ordinary 'every-day' people say with a huge 'can-do' facial expression, that's the baby for me! Advert over and back to watching Coronation Street, the next step having caught the imagination of the would-be athlete and lured by the vision of euphoria ensures people all over the country excitedly comment *'whatever she/he's on I want some! HOW MUCH? £2,000* (and the rest) and with a 'cheap at the price' comment it's – 'I'll have two and on prime time delivery, yahoo and yippee –can't wait, where's my leotard?!!!

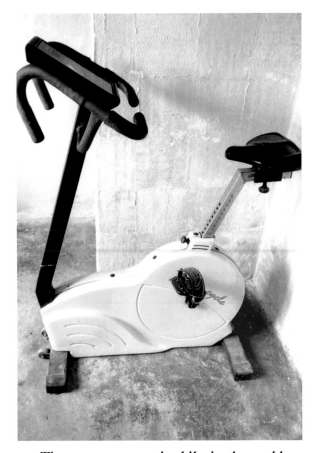

The most unattractive bike in the world

23 years ago I paid £110 for this second-hand bike, yet it has played a major part in my 80 cycling wins – You don't need expensive equipment to be successful!

In all my considerable years as an athlete and professional health and fitness and martial arts exponent, working with Britain's elite fighting force, the Royal Marines, then in three different Sports Centres and with Northumbria Police as a civilian trainer for 24 years, while delivering an array of physical fitness sessions (I'm talking thousands), and within a multitude of formats, including classroom educational sessions, as well as activities of hands-on personal safety or martial arts, there was one word that could (and indeed did) give me nightmares – the word? INJURY! For to lose just one person due to injury from a catchment of hundreds (if not thousands) meant, cessation of exercise and even official training for the individual, and a colossal amount of work for me designed to explain just how the cop (while with Northumbria Police) could not return to frontline duties, and of course even without the spoken word, the 'insinuation' or assumption was that as the supervisor (if not me then one of my trainers) I was somehow negligent! In today's 2021 sporting 'arenas', I would additionally perhaps be found guilty of the poor fellow's developing 'mental health' problems, resulting from the cessation of exercise; I mean nothing could be worse, could it – although the 'athlete' was 10 stones overweight if you get my drift! The latter could well result in internal enquiries and even a trip to court. For to lose a cop due to injury during my 24 years as a Senior Self-Defence Trainer (responsible for a team of six trainers), Physical Training Instructor, or even as referred to by some – Sports Development Officer – during a fairly vigorous training session was sacrament to attempted job-related suicide, and it's a compensation culture, based on a nothing to lose principle. The point I make (in a self-confessed, long-winded fashion) is that for the exercise 'supervisor', trainer, or advisor, an oft forgotten 'duty of care' responsibility is ever-present in today's active fitness sessions. As soon as we put a person into physical motion, there is an inherent 'risk' of injury, and if the risk is not managed appropriately through official risk assessments, there will be a hefty monetary price to pay in terms of the 'avoidable' injury. Isn't it strange with injuries, once liability is established, the sum always increases, because somewhat mysteriously the injury doesn't respond to treatment and even gets worse (well wouldn't you just know it?), and 'all the pain and discomfort' leads to sleepless nights for the former 'self-professed athlete' as he/she tosses and turns in an attempt to get 'comfortable' and so the once anticipated 'trivial knock' takes an ever-developing turn for the worse (or better, depending which side you are representing) – of course, leading to the obligatory mental health issues which in turn lead to a catastrophic breakdown in relationships!

Currently GPs in clinics across the land are being severely criticised for locking themselves away behind closed doors as their clientele desperately seek their personalised attention, it seems that everyone in all occupational positions across the country are now 'mingling' as their jobs dictate, but not the GPs. Yet by all accounts there are many on-line fitness sessions going out to the masses without any on-the-shop floor supervision, apart from a 'just copy me' philosophy! I wonder how many sitting room fitness participants have been laid-up with strains, muscular pulls, broken bones etc while attempting to copy the foreign activities dealt out by the superbly fit presenters, who by all accounts are making quite a bit of money. One of the biggest victories for me in the thousands of fitness and martial art type activities I delivered over many decades was to have everyone leave the session as they started it – injury free!

Back to those 'frenetic' **adverts**. They suggest that the flat-out anaerobic exercises they portray are an everyday joy and something to look forward to as you stir from the cosy comfort of your warm bed every morning. I've never promised anything in this book and never would, because it would be dishonest to do so, there's no guarantee, but I'll get close here, and the promise 'almost' is that the 'harder' and more intense the perceived or anticipated exercise is THE LESS YOU WILL LOOK FORWARD TO IT! For many of us, 'pain' and undue stress is a big de-motivator. Sooner or later, you will wake up and say 'oh to hell, not this morning!' and once you miss that first workout it will give you licence to miss another. Athletes are different, by the way, because their incentive is different, they are way past the 'keep fit' stage, the latter maintenance phase has been replaced by a desire to pit themselves against other 'athletes', and under normal circumstances the incentive that propels them on is 'competition'; however, even athletes need regular amounts of immense will-power to continually beat themselves up during their anaerobic training. For the 'athlete', anaerobic training is as close as it gets to race-type effort – your body is working close to its maximum tolerance, and the effort mimics the intense physical efforts given when trying to defeat other 'gladiators!' By the way, unlike the models, athletes normally don't do more the two or three anaerobic sessions in their seven-day training week, and the intensity of those work-outs will suffer if the athletes' 'aerobic' (stamina/strength) capacity is not first class. Stamina base training for the athlete will always precede the harder/ faster sessions. As I've said many times, *you can't fake stamina, most fit people can sprint 100 metres at least once, but how many can repeat the activity many times – very few – and the few are those who have developed that all-important crucial stamina base.*

With most things in life, you begin with a menu, and the menu offers a choice; for example, enter a restaurant and you'll be handed a menu of available food and drink. Likewise, enter a garage forecourt and you'll sooner rather than later be joined by a salesperson enquiring what sort of vehicle you have in mind. When talking exercise, you also have a menu! Let's take a look.

AEROBIC ACTIVITY

As soon as you move the heart sees a green light and begins work!

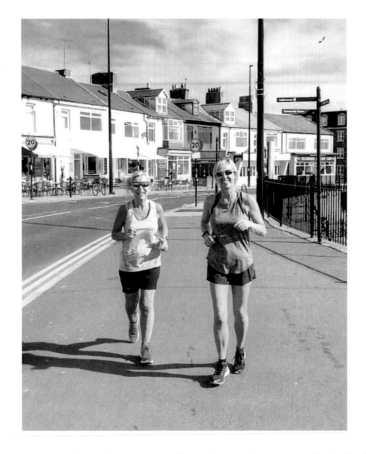

Exercise and smiles from Gill and Lindsay, it can't be bad!

The word 'aerobic' means 'with oxygen', and aerobic activity is exercising whereby the body's demand for oxygen is met during the activity. Aerobic activity is a 'vital' component of physical exercise, so what exactly is aerobic activity?

Just like our car needs an energy supply, in its case petrol, to transport us around, when we exercise we also need an energy supply which enables us to move around – the energy for us comes from two main sources, both circulated and supplied in our blood supply:

1. Nutrients - in the form of the food and drink we consume;
2. Oxygen – taken from the air we breathe.

And if we don't get sufficient of either (energy or oxygen), our ability to sustain the exercise is substantially reduced. Aerobic exercise is performed because the body's demand for oxygen is being met during the physical activity or, in simple terms, we exercise but the extent of the exercise doesn't cause excessive breathlessness, which in turn would slow us down or stop us. If we drive a car at 100mph, incorporating severe stops and accelerating starts, it will very soon exhaust the vehicle's energy supply, in other words to drive it like that is costly, it's not economical (as well as potentially damaging the vehicle's mechanical components etc). However, if we drive slower and therefore conserve the fuel, we can go on for much longer periods whilst also providing longevity for the car's moving components, so aerobic exercise is similar to the latter mode, its 'slower' and 'steady state', or even to a degree rhythmic. When working out aerobically, our pulse rate (derived from the heart, i.e. a heartbeat) can be used as a guide to monitor the rate of effort, a little like the speed monitor on the car console. And so, in simplistic terms, when operating aerobically, the exercise aim is to keep the speed or pace, i.e. while you're walking or running, fairly constant throughout, as opposed to a fluctuation as occurs for example during short sharp hard bursts of activity such as repeated sprints or the lifting of heavy weights or maybe in a judo competition.

What can I hope to gain by Aerobic exercise?

It's my oft considered opinion, and despite the continuous coming and going of 'trends', no other form of exercise plays such a crucial role in the maintenance of the body, through basic exercise physiology and therefore general health as does aerobic activity, and that's because amongst other elements it exercises the cardio-vascular system, the engine room of the human body.

It is generally accepted that the heart, lungs and circulatory system (often collectively referred to as the cardio-vascular system or cardio-respiratory system) is an immensely important area when discussing general health and fitness. This being the case, careful consideration should be given to its maintenance. If the heart stops or malfunctions in any way, then life itself is at risk. The heart is but a muscle whose sole purpose in life is to keep us alive; it performs this function by circulating blood around the body with every beat it delivers, and as mentioned previously, in the blood we have oxygen from the air we breathe and we have energy derived from our intake of food and drink. If the cardiovascular system works well, the everyday physical side of life is generally a 'doddle', i.e. going to work, running after a bus, climbing stairs, washing the car, gardening, housework or whatever causes no real concern. However, if the cardio-vascular system becomes inefficient, i.e. the heart (a muscle) becomes weak and flabby, due in the main to a lack of physical activity and maybe an inappropriate diet, then all physical activity can become abnormally difficult as well as mentally stressful. This leads to an early onset of fatigue, undue breathlessness and possibly dizziness in the short term and ultimately a big reduction in your capacity to perform what were once simple everyday physical tasks in the long term.

How can I do aerobic exercise?

Your own personal fitness condition at the time of beginning an exercise programme, together with any known ailments, will generally dictate which exercises you choose. Your choice should include a lot of common sense, and some thought should also be given to your current physical stature.

Some aerobic activities are substantially weight-bearing, so for example, if you are 5' 2" tall and weigh 15 stones, running would be a poor choice (until, that is, you substantially reduce your weight). The stress you would put on your skeletal frame in this instance would invariably result in some form of injury, which obviously defeats the object.

Before we look at some of the forms of available exercise, here is a bit of cautionary advice which we should all consider 'before' your main exercise choice. Remember, and I can't stress this enough, longevity is perhaps the most important aim, so warm-up well, and make the session manageable.

Mobility and flexibility

(including warm-ups and cool-downs)

With everything in life there is a start, middle, and an end; with physical exercise, the start should always incorporate the often mundane but very important warm-up procedure. We all have an individual range of movement which will vary from person to person. When we exercise, that range of movement immediately increases and lengthens, i.e. your stride length if jogging increases substantially more than that of walking. It is also accepted that some of us can reach or stretch further than others, although our height and general physical stature may well be similar. Our ability to stretch (range of movement) is governed to a certain degree by genetic factors and age; some people are born more flexible than others and generally speaking females and children are more flexible than males and adults, but with care you can increase your range of movement and with the improvements, reduce the potential of injury whilst extending stride length in running or range of movement in the water.

There is little doubt that poor flexibility resulting in a poor range of movement (upper body and lower limbs) may result in 'injury' problems in the form of strains and muscle pulls. Furthermore, the older we become quite naturally through the aging process, the less agile we may become; however, as with so many issues age need not be a total negative or an excuse – if it's important you work at it!

Regular stretching exercises performed safely can substantially increase our range of movement and in the process help in the prevention of injuries. Stretching exercises systematically performed as part of your 'warm-up' prior to exercise and again following exercise, that's during your 'cool-down', is an uncomplicated method of achieving and maintaining improvement in this area.

Warm-ups

It could be argued that the initial warm-up is the most important part of any training session or competition. *I had students at work who quite regularly would ask if they could miss the warm-up on the basis that the energy used to prepare may detract from their timed assessment, ha! My response was always the same: the warm-up* is *designed to assist in your assessment or workout, not to inhibit it.* Time spent 'preparing' to exercise or compete allows the body and the mind to tune in to the approaching rigours of the activity. In the current world with all its 'ifs' and 'buts' and the never ending analysis of 'everything', as mentioned above, if someone was injured during a supervised session, there is little doubt I would have had to write in detail the warm-up procedure I had used, and once the familiar time consuming 'claim' for compensation had landed on my desk from the student, their physical injury would have no doubt multiplied due to their sleepless nights, stress, as well as the ongoing and persistent pain – talk about 'working the system'! Being the occasional cynic I can be, I often thought people only came to the gym or training so they could go sick afterwards, have a couple of weeks off, and if they were really ambitious top up their forthcoming holiday spending money following their anticipated claim! Anyhow, warm-ups are crucial and are designed to assist the person, not to detract from their efforts.

A gradual warm-up process should pre-empt all energetic activities to simply prepare our bodies for 'action' – see below.

In line with this current chapter, and a practical example. **How 'not' to start a Park Run!** At Park Runs (see Park Runs chapter) people often arrive at the very last minute, and as such their warm-up begins and ends with a sprint from the car to the start vicinity. Subsequently, at the off there is an immediate rush of blood to energise the body, and breathlessness follows quickly afterwards to compensate the sudden energy surge, as the body tries its best to meet the hurried demands placed on it by the participant. My own warm-ups follow a well-rehearsed procedure along the following lines: For Park Runs I begin by walking for 10 minutes before the start to gently warm my body and gently stretch my legs; after 10 minutes or so I begin to jog slowly, in the process gradually elevating my heart rate as the body warms, then I warm up muscle tissue and prepare tendons for the more vigorous efforts that will follow; after 10-15minutes, depending on the air temperature (the colder the weather, the more I warm-up), I'll walk for a few minutes and then begin a basic stretching routine. There are various ways to stretch; these include: *Static stretching* is performed slowly and gradually and is whereby the person applies the stretch and holds it still (without jerking) for several seconds i.e. 20-45s. Ballistic stretching is bouncing-type movements and may present a greater risk of injury if not performed carefully and in line with the person's capabilities. Dynamic stretches are often used to replicate the person's sporting movement i.e. arm circles as in swimming front crawl. It's all about preparing the body for the forthcoming activity, so you stretch those areas which you will be using during the activity. On a personal basis, I go systematically, head to toe, doing the legs last. So, head, neck, shoulders and arms, hips, groin, thighs, hamstrings (back of legs) and finally calves, feet. For upper body I do ballistic stretches (arm swings), for legs I do mainly 'static' stretching whereby you gradually extend the range of movement then hold each stretch for 20-30 seconds. Now, stretching for the Park Runs shouldn't hurt, but there will be some slight discomfort as the muscles and tendons gradually adapt and lengthen. Once stretching is over, I then walk again to keep warm and shake things loose. Then I jog and finally I do some faster efforts, e.g. 10 x 50 metre strides with walk back between, then jog and walk for the final 10 minutes before the off. Once again there are literally numerous ways of getting both your body and mind in a good place, so if you need to, take the above method simply as a guide. If I'm doing a triathlon, I work systematically the other way round, that is leaving the upper body till last as the arms, shoulders and chest have the greatest stress at the beginning with the swimming being the first of the three disciplines. Makes sense? And back to Aerobic activities.

Cool Downs

In brief, a cool-down is the reverse of the warm-up. The warm-up gradually prepares the body for more intense exercise, the cool-down takes the body gradually from where it was after your efforts to where it was before the commencement of exercise, although in the warm-up the activities go from little to more, for the cool-down we then go in the other direction from more intense exercise to less. So we warm-up to prepare the body for the activities about to happen, while cool-downs help to gradually take the body back to where it was at the beginning, so jog slowly, stretch, put on warm clothing and begin the replenishing process (fuel including liquid), cool-downs help to prevent 'blood pooling' (see page x) and assist in the elimination of wastes which built up during the exercise and stagnating within blood vessels and muscles after the exercise. Cool-downs gradually return you back to normal mode.

There was a short article in today's paper from a Science Correspondent, advising us that – Watering the roses is 'as good as a gym session' (I knew what he meant by the way, mental 'well-being' and all that). Apparently, the more you garden, the better the outcome. I knew a physio once who hated the springtime, because all his clientele were older gardeners – out of hibernation, and now seeking treatment from the effects of their 'sudden' gardening activities – mmm! The scientist (above) went on to say the impact of gardening had the same positive outcome as vigorous exercises such as running and cycling. Even if there is some merit in the results of that presumed experiment, not everyone has a garden, but tell you what we do have – **SHOES!**

WALKING!

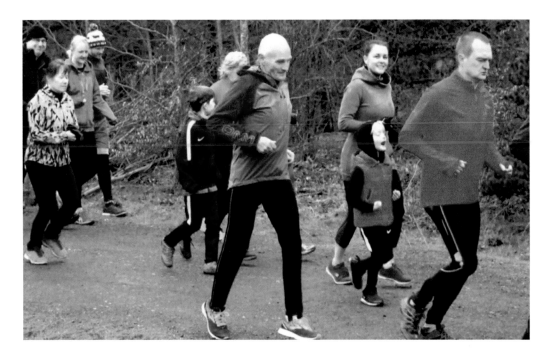

"If you can talk while exercising, it's fair to say you are working aerobically, here's young Dan and his Mam singing 'Nellie keep ya bellie close to mine' Who taught him that?

It's a great place to start! And perhaps the one and only instinctive exercise we can do almost forever – now that's the *longevity* I keep harping on about!

Don't scoff at the activity of walking; after all, it's a very energetic and competitive Olympic sport! Walking is the most natural of all physical exercises – as babies the urge to leave crawling behind on the living room carpet and get up onto two feet is as normal and as instinctive as filling our nappies! Walking, even as babes, requires no coaching; in contrast, swimming does, cycling does, aerobic dance and so many other activities do, but not walking. Furthermore, use regular walking as a means of remaining physically active, and unlike many other activities you'll do it for the remainder of your life. As adults, *'how'* we walk is fundamental in terms of improving (or even maintaining) our general fitness. My observations are that most people don't walk quickly enough, many of us dawdle and for many others our body alignment is poor, being slumped over with a curvature of the spine and shuffling as opposed to being upright and striding out is common. In order to make gains aerobically, slow walking should be looked upon as merely a 'warm-up' exercise which precedes 'faster' meaningful walking; as a guide a comment such as *'Sorry, I'll see you later, I'm in a hurry'*, is a good principle which may enable you to bring some 'quality' into the activity of walking.

During my time in the Royal Marines, 'walking' (not sprinting) was at the heart of almost everything we did. I can 'almost' recall (as a 16 year old) the last week of our 16-week 'Commando Training' down at Lympstone (which followed on from 32 weeks of 'basic' training at Deal) and to successfully pass-out with the iconic, coveted Green Beret placed firmly on our proud heads, and alongside other physical competencies we had Endurance Courses, Assault Courses, the appropriately named Tarzan Course, a 9-mile Speed March **(see page x)** all culminating with a 30-mile timed route march on Dartmoor – all were completed in full fighting equipment and all were timed. We learned to walk with just about the same pace as many run, and it's the pace of the activity which carries most 'Brownie' points from the cardio perspective, slow methodical sluggish loitering will have limited rewards, and not give you the same benefits as fast walking will. Now if you are capable of 'fast' or 'brisk' walking – who's to say you can't gradually bring slow jogging into your life? Even if it is interspersed with brisk walking.

There are countless contradictions on exercise, and 'one man's meat', as the saying goes 'is another's poison'. What works for one is contrary to another, and with all exercises, there are pros and cons. While discussing walking in particular, it is 'safe', it can be done almost anywhere, it needs minimal support equipment and there are few risks. However, to benefit from it (and I accept fully this is obvious) you need to focus on elevating your heart rate (HR). All physical training is based on the *'overload'* principle – in simplistic terms all that means is for your body to allow positive changes to take place and improve, in terms of physical efficiency you need to work it above its normal range. As an example: if your resting pulse rate (while sitting down), is 70 beats per minute*, and your walking heart rate is the same as your resting heart rate (unlikely but ...!) there is no cardio-vascular stimulus present to overload the system. The overload is required to kickstart a physiological improvement process. If your walking is designed as a 'keep fit' or 'get fitter' exercise you should tax yourself over the resting norm, whilst working within safe or comfortable limits, upping your breathing rate, whilst not causing 'pain' – remember we call this aerobic conditioning – with oxygen, not without oxygen. So a basic easy to understand practical example based on a resting HR of 70bpm would be: Begin walking at a comfortable pace (e.g. 80/90bpm), with good body position; after approximately five minutes consciously walk a bit faster (HR 110bpm), then depending on your fitness level and your aim elevate it again (e.g. 120bpm) by consciously increasing your pace and therefore your effort; therein lies the 'overload' principle which is essential to improved fitness. In conclusion: if your body is working harder, well, it requires more fuel, and the fuel is provided by your heart's pumping action which circulates more blood around the body and in so doing satisfying the muscles with the oxygen and nutrition it needs (fuel) to satisfy the demands deriving from the exercise. As a guide, regarding suitable effort levels, the 'talk test' can be useful, which simply means – if you can reasonably hold a conversation with your dog while walking (if Rover can't reply – you may need to slow, for the poor little canine) you are working out aerobically. If you are struggling to say 'sit', then slow down, ease up and drop your efforts and with it your HR.

> *People's resting heart rate can vary substantially; by and large (providing you have no underlying health issues) the lower it is whilst sitting comfortably at ease and stress-free, the more efficient it is, simply indicating the pump is doing more work for less effort with each beat, because it is fit and strong. A couple of nights ago mine was 45 bpm, now when I was at my peak it was as low as 36/7 bpm, nothing at all to brag about, of course, just fact.

Tell you what, though, although the above principles are simple and easy to verbally explain, 'just try writing them down in a readable non-complex way, it's not so easy!' I can remember years ago being given a punishment at school for some sort of wrongdoing (I'd be totally innocent –of course) and the punishment was writing down the 'Lord's Prayer' in its entirety! We rhymed it daily, and at other times as we waited to be caned, but writing it down had us in all sorts of trouble – in fact getting the cane would have been kinder.

If you read the information on interval training, fartlek training, etc. somewhere in this Aerobic chapter you can use those same principles whilst making your walking 'training' more interesting and more productive.

Some additional key aerobic activities are listed shortly but finding a form of exercise you are comfortable with should be the priority. Variety as they say is the spice of life and it is beneficial to vary your exercise routine (see chapter on Cross Training); in so doing you will shift the emphasis from one body part to another which in turn will assist in the recovery process. So, a simple 'example' could read – jog on a Monday, do some upper-body weights on a Tuesday, swim on Wednesdays, go for a walk on Thursday etc. The principle of this is simple and is a great way to ensure recovery whilst still being able to exercise in some way. It's important to mention that you don't have to exercise every day – taking the occasional day off is not a sin! Although 'consistency' should be the aim, if you don't see improvement after a month or so (and sometimes you get worse, due to the un-accustomed exercise stress, before you get better) review both your choice of activity, your degree of effort and how long you perform it for, e.g. if you're struggling with a five-mile cycle ride the 'journey' may be too long, or if the 'effort is not taxing enough or too easy the 'training effect' may also be delayed. Remember to listen to your heart rate as a guide – as a tentative guide take your resting pulse i.e. from 70 or 80 beats per minute up to 100-140 bpm. *The latter is simply a guide; we're all different, try not to compare too much with someone else who is perhaps working alongside you.*

Blood Pooling (worth a mention)

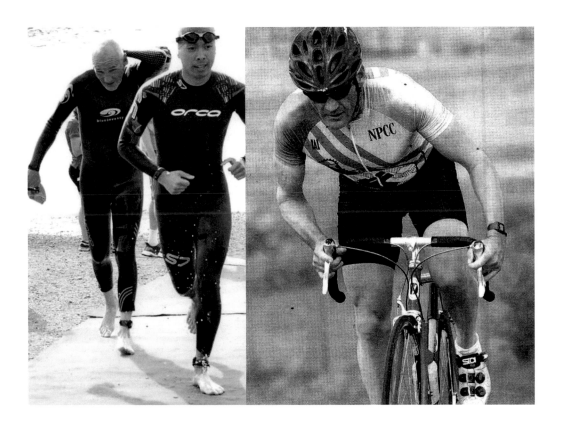

Different types of exercise require different amounts of blood to fuel the body, so swimming is mainly upper body and cycling is mainly lower body – Hence the term 'blood pooling'.

As mentioned previously in this aerobic section, the body's 'fuel' is a mixture of oxygen and nutrients, the body has a highway, consisting of the engine (heart) which pumps blood along the highway to various destinations. Once you begin to exercise, the demand for fuel increases and is immediate; the harder the exercise the more fuel required (just like your vehicle – the faster you drive the more petrol you burn). Blood (via the heart) is used to transfer the two commodities. If I step, run or cycle, then the legs (thighs and calves) require most of the fuel, so the blood makes the transfer – wonderful, isn't it, no mobiles required! If I swim then the upper body (shoulders, arms and back) needs and receives most blood. *Blood pooling* occurs when one part of the body receives more blood than another. In terms of triathlon, when I come out of the water after the swim, my upper body is blood 'heavy', I run up the slope from the swim to the bike transition and my legs may for a short period feel strangely weak because there is a time delay before the blood will circulate to my legs. It happens the same way in your first aid course, if a heart attack has occurred or if someone has fainted, we're advised to lie the casualty down and raise their legs which helps facilitate oxygen carrying blood to the heart, assisting in the recovery procedure! Although it sounds minor, and it is to a degree, that's why I have different warm-up procedures for differing activities. We'll have a look at diet soon; however, that's why eating and drinking too close to exercise is also not recommended (because the blood is working hard in the digestive system at that time). *Isn't the body just the most incredible automatic bit of kit on the planet?*

Additional Aerobic Activities

(I'd be here forever if I was to explain them all in detail, so the following is for your perusal only. What they should share common ground with is the effect on Heart Rate – 'steady state' allowing for continuity!)

You have a wide choice. Faster walking, as above (remember you are trying to increase your heart rate), hill walking, dancing, jogging (e.g. eight to 11 minute miles), running (six to eight minutes per mile and faster), rowing, swimming, stepping, skiing, cycling, some forms of class aerobics, steady state circuit training etc. The problem with 'classes' and 'groups' is derived from numbers, and it's likely that there will be a wide variety of conditions within the group, so be prepared to abort a bit early depending on how you are coping! There's no shame in that, and as far as I'm concerned, it's a token of your intelligence.

For beginners, as a general guide, the basic aim should be to exercise reasonably comfortably for approximately 20 minutes. It should be a steady pace with the pulse rate normally between approximately 100 and 140 beats per minute (that is just a guide and don't become obsessed by pulse rates), depending on your current physical condition, past history and your age.

Pulse monitors can be relatively cheap and provide interesting data; apart from exercising, your heart rate (just like your blood pressure) will naturally vary at certain times, depending on what you're doing or even thinking. To get reasonably correct averages, take the pulse at the same times every few days. If you weigh yourself then mornings straight from bed are best.

Although I have suggested sessions of 20 minutes to gain the desired training effect and to noticeably see improvement, it may take several weeks or even months to progress to this level – so be patient. I cannot stress enough the importance of consistency (three-four times a week is fine – and based on the guidelines above that's barely an hour to 80 minutes in the week and there's 168 hours to choose from!).

Digressing for a moment, as you do in occasional discussions – and CONSIDER THE FOLLOWING!

It is currently fashionable to make the subject of health, and exercise in particular, a complex science, and the more complex the subject appears, well the more you pay – right? For many health and fitness exponents, it's a business, an opportunity not to be missed to make a bob or two, and as such there is a constant bombardment of ever-changing information available primarily by using the media as the distribution point.

'Research and studies' – give me a break!!

Someone somewhere must be making a lot of money by using the repetitive mantra of the word – **Research!!!!!** The latter singular word accompanies some famed and 'noted' so called 'celebrity experts' and Newspaper Columnists 'everywhere'. 'All' their regular published articles and weekly newspaper columns commence (just like 'Our Father' precedes the Lord's Prayer) with the words – *'Recent research has indicated'* before the expert puts on a learned mantle and attempts to transfer the 'new' research into a readable format that the reader can at least partially understand. Following the acquisition of the new info, the reader, for the most part, will change little, if at all; last week's 'recent research has indicated' article is now resigned to history. My personal gripe is, that once 'today's' newly acquired research (and there'll be some more tomorrow) has been deciphered and interpreted into a readable format by the wealthy non-participating 'expert', then the findings have surely got to offer something of a 'practical benefit' to the eager reader other than filling another newspaper column using information carried out in the confines of a laboratory! My own view is that, in terms of physical fitness or improved nutrition, any new research dispensed from the lab has got to be acquirable or available from either the Co-op's food-laden shelves, or from the practicality of being able to physically partake in the newly discovered and magical exercise routine. Experienced practitioners in all things, at least in principle, have so much more to offer that those clothed in white overalls or neatly pressed suits accompanied by reams of statistics housed in briefcases. What I mean is, if you want to learn how to swim don't go to Google and type in 'recent research into swimming'; instead go take a lesson or two from an experienced swimming teacher. Likewise, if you want to know the best way to begin a running programme tailor-made just for you, don't purchase an expensive 'scientific approach to running' manual authored by a doctor with a degree in ? – instead go to the Morpeth Harriers for a bit of 'practical' advice from their experienced coaches (who do the coaching for fun – not money)and not to your slightly overweight General Practitioner sitting comfortably in your local clinic, because the GP is likely to do exactly what the newspaper columnist does and that is google 'recent findings into practical running'!

Four terms used every five minutes at the moment, which are clearly intended to help sell the authors' books and the programme presenters' fitness manuals etc. are: **'research has indicated' OR 'studies have shown', OR 'based on scientific analysis', OR 'recent trials have revealed'; the words repetitively accompany all information on health and fitness and the above terms are guaranteed a place within all, you name it, newspapers, books, television presentations, and magazine supplements, all that is except mine. At 70** years of age, I rarely need them, and I most certainly wouldn't buy them. As a species, the human-form has remained pretty much the same for centuries; however, the 'data' handed down from the experiments changes like the weather, over the years there has been a lot of 'inconsistency' in relation to new research.

Here's a thing, for as long as you and I have been kicking around there has been 'research' and there has been 'studies' – presumably it keeps people in work. It seems to me that if 'new' studies and 'new' research are to be believed and accepted as correct, then all the countless 'old studies' and 'old research' we've been handed, must have been false, although of course you'd expect that the earlier 'research' and 'studies' would have had the same intense scrutiny, and been subjected to the same meticulously researched and studied subjects as that given to the new stuff! That being a logical assumption just made by the former Royal Marine who's sitting here without a degree in sports science, but with a seriously furrowed brow whilst musing over this enigma. Now think about this. On the latter principle, it must also be fair to say, that the 'newer' research and studies that'll be given 'tomorrow' will also mean that the research and studies conducted and given 'today' must also be just waiting to be declared as wrong, otherwise why replace it! Somewhat refreshingly perhaps is that the vast majority of my views are derived through personal 'trial and error' and persistent non-stop hours spent as a 'practitioner' in the health and fitness subjects, as well as an everyday accomplished Athlete, as well as a certified Trainer, Teacher, Coach and Instructor operating within the working environment; as a bonus, I've also won 'big' championships on the back of my knowledge. At the risk of repeating myself (I've said it before), the last comments don't make me right, of course, and who knows, maybe if I'd adhered to all the differing professional scientific advice coming in from the Laboratories, the Doctors and Professors I'd have performed better – too late now to find out – but without any of it, I did pretty good. AND I'm still doing pretty good, decades later, and there's a boat load of scientific advice that's gone soaring past me in swathes of water under my bridges. Let me say this, the latter, somewhat quirky views and comments are based purely on 'common-sense' (there is some history in the latter 'common-sense' theme – I once was the proud recipient of a huge cup given to the Royal Marine showing the most initiative in 'expedition training'. The latter's not a degree in sports science, of course, nevertheless!). I sincerely hope the expressed views have not resulted in me sounding in any way pompous, arrogant or even dare I say clever, regardless, the following details are self-explanatory.

I am today, 70 years old, having walked the dog for 45 minutes, ran six miles in the snow and ice, followed immediately by 90 minutes on my ancient rusty static bike, and some stretching to conclude. I have all my own teeth (bar two, and those two have let me down big style, the gits!), my blood pressure is 114/69, I have a resting heart rate today of 47 bpm, my weight is constant at 10st 3lbs (my fighting weight when at my athletic peak 40years ago) which was my weight when I was winning 47 triathlons and many British titles in the 1980s/90s and a former British Ironman record holder. Similarly, before that, I was racing and winning marathons in the 1970s against 'athletes' during the 'running boom'. Today, like most days, I have no notable aches and pains (although my wife says I audibly creak occasionally – so maybe my hearing is 'normal'), my knees are wonderful as are my hips, and that's also taking into account that between the ages of 50 and 60 I won at least 75 open cycle races (those results 'weren't' age-group related, I was beating others half my age). And today I can't wait to get out of this so frustrating Covid lockdown so I can resume my triathlons, cycle races, playing with a band, and racing around Park Runs where I am still standing on the front line in front of hundreds, because my finishing positions allow me to. Now the latter aren't guesswork, they are fact. So, based on where I've been, and where I am today, I must be doing something right; additionally I do it all so differently from the advice derived from the 'research' and 'studies'-have-indicated crew!!

Here's another contradiction that goes against the grain: I've never in my whole life 'slept well' (I am a real pain to sleep with, although I do 'try oh so hard'). I continue to try hard simply because I am being consistently and reliably told if I don't get to sleep soon, well, I'll have mental health issues resulting in dementia possibly as early as Monday next, so with that advice, I'd better sleep well tonight then – help! The enigma is: does someone giving you the above 'helpful' information really help you sleep better? I think not – 'do you?' Better take 'some more' pills then, eh? Or have a word with the 'sleep expert' to see what the research says. An 'advert' I saw last night re getting a good night's sleep ended with a quiet warning – 'read the label' and 'don't take for more than two weeks' – now there's a cause for concern that'll keep me up all night, if ever you've heard one! Might do some 'pre-sleeping exercises' (then I'll keep Jen up as well!). For 40 years I never took so much as a single aspirin, codeine, or paracetamol! Enough! Let's move on, but before that a small piece of personal history!

When I was a kid, I can remember shouting through the bedroom wall, 'what time is it, Mam?' and she would shout back 'It's 2 o'clock, now for god's sake go to sleep or you'll not get up for school!'. But you know what? I always did get up for school, never missed a shift – 100% attendance always, still got the end of term books! For 24 years with my last employer, never so much as a single day's absence! Later in life, my mother, as always, had a non-complex common sense view on the latter: 'Michael you were always excited about something, son, that's why sleep was ever elusive – I could have murdered you!!!'

Training principles are not complex, although timing and peaking for special events can be!

If we systematically, progressively and regularly exercise the body over and above what it would normally do in the course of an average day, it will adapt and react by becoming more efficient and stronger and maybe even quicker within the areas worked. For example, if we do biceps curls, then we increase the efficiency and the working capacity of the bicep muscles; if we likewise exercise aerobically, then we increase the working capacity of the cardio-vascular system.

Rest and recovery!

It is very important to realise that training is a destructive process. Whilst working out we not only deplete energy stores in the form of sugars and fat (depending on the type of exercise), but we also break down muscle tissue. Physical improvement does not take place during the exercise, it takes place during the rest periods following the exercise, so we must allow sufficient rest and recovery between sessions, otherwise, far from improving our physical state, we may end up being continually run down, tired, or worse again injured.

Is it working?

Exercising aerobically is a good method of burning body fat (as an energy source) – you don't see many fat marathon runners or Tour de France riders. If you combine aerobic workouts with a reduction in your calorie intake, you should see some reduction in body weight; now that's just common sense. Also, as your cardio- vascular system becomes more efficient through regular exercise, your resting pulse rate should become noticeably slower, indicating your heart is performing the same workload as before but with less effort due to its increased strength and improving efficiency. Pulse taking is made even easier by the host of watches currently available.

A word of caution (sorry, it goes with the subject!)

If you have a known medical ailment or your family has a history of a medical condition, if you are overweight or have led (up to now) a predominantly sedentary lifestyle, if you smoke or have smoked in the past and generally often feel 'unwell', it makes sense to have a quick MOT (medical check-up) with your GP prior to beginning your exercise programme. This will take about 10-15 minutes of your time and invariably give you peace of mind.

One thing that's always bothered me after writing and speaking on health and fitness issues is tempting fate! If I die soon (maybe I'm found lying in a field somewhere smiling, probably with a protective hand or two cupping my nuts) I hereby give you the absolute right, nay I 'order' you, to have a bloody good side splitting laugh till the tears trickle down your rosy red cheeks whilst muttering 'here's Harris, the git, feeding us all that crap on brown bread and apples and doesn't he just go and die on us, ha ha ha – mine's a Guinness, no make that two – I'll drink his as well! As Jennifer quietly mutters 'trust him – he'll have done it on purpose, and that grass needs cut'!

To Jim Taylor and my Uncle Robert: I visit Jim weekly (when Covid allows), he's currently 92 and a great 'crack'. Jim's best friend was my Uncle Robert, they grew up together in the Northumbrian pit village of Radcliffe before joining the Black Watch together; Robert was like me, a Physical Training Instructor. In later life Robert 'caught' Alzheimer's (hope it wasn't off me) and myself and Jim were his only real Care Home visitors. Jim would take Robert to Warkworth in his car for ice cream. And I would take Robert some decent clothes including a Great Britain tracksuit. One lovely spring morning I collected him from his Care Home with the intention of going for a leisurely walk in the warm sunshine and smell the bluebells. As the two of us 'marched' down the long straight Widdrington village road, Robert (resplendent in his GB tracksuit), without any notice 'took off' straight into a sprint, knees almost touching his chest, arms pumping like a windmill. Momentarily stunned and so slow out of the blocks, I ran after him; can you see us? We were both laughing hysterically as cars sped past peeping their horns, drivers no doubt saying 'that old guy must have escaped!' – God only knows what the two of us must have looked like. Once caught up, we both slowed down and looked at each other, him no doubt wondering 'who the hell I was'! Robert's last run will never be forgotten. Jim, thank you so much, my friend, for both your personal friendship and above all your loyalty to your best mate and my Unc! It's not PC, but sod it – the two of you were/are men's men, hard, funny, and with a degree of chivalry!

ENDEAVOUR WE CONQUER

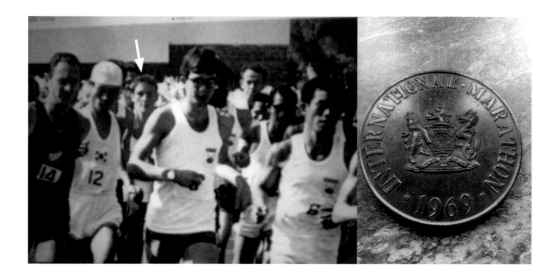

My first marathon, having just turned 18, was a race with a huge difference from the norm because it was ran on very little specific training and fuelled in a fine hotel dining room in the Far-East by bacon, eggs, sausage, mushrooms, beans, fried bread and a nice cuppa tea! Additionally on offer in this hotel there was some 'oh so attractive' and rarely seen soft velvet pink, no slip, toilet paper, can you imagine? Whoopee! What Joy! Hooray! Enough to make you sing and dance! And wait for it, you could use as much of the roll as you liked! You don't believe me, do you? Neither did boys back at 40 Commando! Until I took a roll out of my bag, and piece by piece shared it around!

During a recent phone conversation with my Royal Marine buddy Tommy Gunning, I was reminded about a marathon I did many years ago in 1969 in Hong Kong when I was barely 18 years of age. Tommy, with an uncanny mind for detail had carried out a bit of research into this event and came up with an interesting statistic which was that there were just 28 of us specifically invited 'International' starters in this inaugural event back in 1969 and now fast forward 51 years later to 2020 and the same, now annual marathon, and there were one or two more entries amounting to – wait for it – 75,000 starters!

Keeping it brief, and without going into too much unnecessary detail, I was somewhat strangely present for this occasion and taking part in this special race purely on the rather daft incomprehensible Monty Python type basis that I'd recently won the Royal Navy/Royal Marine Cross Country Championship in Singapore (a four-mile somewhat lumpy race, which was over within 22 minutes). At the time of this event, I had been operationally drafted to the Far East joining 40 Commando Unit, Royal Marines in Singapore for an 18-month stint which entailed regularly moving in and out of the hostile Malaysian Jungle while participating in 'Jungle Warfare' training! Anyhow, after that Championship win I was approached by a rather smart uniformed Naval Lieutenant Commander who asked me *if I'd like to go to Hong Kong and run a race*. Ha ha, you bet I would, 'sir', whoopee, can you imagine? Even now 50 odd years later and I can hardly write for laughing! I mean, would I like to what? – Out of the jungle and onto an exotic airliner with proper cushioned seats, bound for Hong Kong, and polite smiling female air hostesses in starched uniforms, a hint of aftershave and little hats! I'm slavering! I mean as close as I'd been before to anything remotely similar was doing 'eagle flights' while flying in Royal Navy Helicopters many hazardous feet off the ground, with impatient, rough and ready naval crew pushing us hastily out of the juddering chopper doors of a noisy Wessex whilst the ever-present smell of poop mingled amongst us, before rolling around on the unruly tangled undergrowth of a hostile jungle landscape. Now, as is universally known, 'I ain't very bright (even my nana was heard to remark to my concerned mother after a shockingly inept school report *'you can't get blood out of a stone, Margaret'*), so even without too many of the event's details, even I wasn't going to say 'no thanks' to such an overly generous offer! I mean, Hong Kong for an anticipated 'jog in the sun', bring it on, baby. And so a short while later I boarded the civilian aircraft and away I went smiling over the blue ocean to Hong Kong. The only problem was that the officer had been talking about a flaming *'Marathon' the scale of which I totally underestimated, it being 26.2 miles (that's 22.2 miles further than my recent cross country win!). Anyhow, a short while later having been put up in a rather grand Hong Kong hotel, with a super duper breakfast and wonderful toilet roll, I stepped onto a running track with 27 other international athletes and proceeded to run the marathon in* 3 hours and 10 minutes in the Hong Kong sun and, I was hit by a car during the race, honestly, but it was all so worth it – despite the, em, *slight discomfort, and bruising!*

Anyhow, on conclusion of my recent conversation with Tommy, I was instinctively drawn to the least viewed trophy cabinet in the whole world (made by Keith the joiner at work) which stands 'off the beaten track' in a shadowy corner of our house and inside propped up against the cabinet wall is this unique big, heavy, solid and rather grand medal (one of 28 in the whole world) inscribed on one side with *Hong Kong International Marathon 1969* and on the other side a rather touching *Endeavour We Conquer inscription*. Must be worth a bob or two now, don't you think?

For athletes, every medal we possess has a very personal story, but this one is perhaps a bit special: Hong Kong, man – a cooked breakfast and soft pink loo roll – and a stunning one-of-a-kind medal!!!

In line with the above – and I'll pounce on the chance to mention a quick word on nutrition, a subject I will cover in more detail soon in this book – in the case of running a marathon at 18 years of age on so little preparation, and on what amounted to a totally inappropriate diet of greasy fat and suspect dubious protein as well as so little in the way of proper fuel that carbohydrates offer, I would say this.

When we are young, we can exist on almost anything in the nutritional sense providing there is enough of it – a young body can quite happily get by while eating and drinking a boat load of nutritional garbage; in fact, teeth will noticeably suffer long before the body begins its decline. However as the young new body ages, things begin to gradually change, and it's a little like repeatedly applying major force onto the brake pedal of a new car – initially, because of the newness of the brake pedal the

extreme 'stomping' practice used to slow the car down works great for a while; however, in time the inappropriate pressure and misuse continually applied to the pedal begins to reduce the car's braking performance, the product wears noticeably and the wearing, of course, begins to inhibit performance. The same principle happens within the human body, filling it up continually with nutritional garbage will result gradually (at first) in decreased performance. In my opinion, what we eat and drink is the most important aspect of everything within the vast subject of promoting positive human health – eat badly, just like misuse of the brake, and you'll inhibit performance, while reducing the prospect of longevity.

At 18 I ran a marathon in 3hrs 10mins fuelled by saturated fat and little else; 10 years later and thereafter while running with Morpeth Harriers I ran all of my six marathons under 2hrs 30mins. At 36 years of age, though, I ran another marathon in 3hours and 21 minutes (that's 11 minutes slower than my first one in Hong Kong) BUT this marathon was the final part of an Ironman Triathlon and before this marathon had even started I had swam 2.4 miles in a cold lake and cycled 112 miles on a hilly course. At 70, I still perform with a degree of distinction; I'm top 5 this year overall, twice from two, and race weekly 10 mile cycling time trials in 23 minutes, I also run, swim and do a variety of strength and flexibility exercises. I believe the main reason for the recent performances over the preceding 10 years, and a continuation of my persistently vigorous life is that my diet is 'sound' and has been for years and years because I keep an ever keen vigilant eye on it. So the internal side (stomach, digestive organs etc.) matches and complements the outside (muscular and skeletal frame). I enthusiastically still exercise and train every day of my life! Please don't confuse the latter statements as some sort of pompous brag, because I revel in declaring regularly that *I'm not at all special, just a very ordinary bloke from the North East!* But, I don't get ill, I've got the vast majority of my original teeth, my cardio is just superb and all my muscles, bones and sinews function just great and still at a premium level (up till now anyway – touch wood eh), and I put so much of the latter down to doing tomorrow what I do today, I truly can't think of another reason! By the way, in finishing this chapter, if I 'kick it' soon, *please have a good laugh,* I mean it, because I've probably had more out of my

70 current years than many others get out of reaching a ton and beyond! You reap what you sow!! I don't owe anything, I cost you nothing, and what I have in all aspects of my life, including health and fitness – I've worked for!

JOGGING and RUNNING!

(I'll keep this as simple as I can)

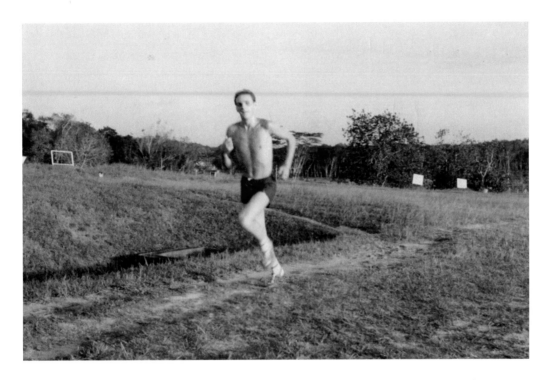

'Sometimes we just happen to be in the right place at just the right time!'

I have often wondered what it must have been like walking around the Mathew Street area of Liverpool in 1961, when an 'unknown' foursome calling themselves **The Beatles** began to emerge on the musical scene and for the first time, turn heads, while playing R&B in an innocuous, dank, sweaty cellar called The Cavern. Or likewise, maybe being around in 1962 when another anonymous musical outfit calling themselves The Rolling Stones got a residency at the Crawdaddy Club in Richmond, Surrey. Or more localised, what about the Hirst Park area of Ashington in Northumberland in the 1950s where Bobby and

Jack Charlton were part of regular Sunday afternoon hastily-arranged football matches which would take them on a footballing journey culminating in the two brothers, who with anther nine teammates, took on and beat the world!

Motivation is just another word in the English dictionary. Yet a word so bristling with importance that it is solely responsible for almost everything we do, yet that singular word is the prompt, the starting nucleus which compels many of us to seek out a life so different from others. And where did the 'spark' that is called motivation initially materialise from?

For me it probably happened in my boarding school, which was situated in the scenic, wild, heather-clad hills around the small Northumbrian village of Bellingham in the summer of 1965. At the time in question, I was being a complete irritating jerk one Saturday afternoon; as such and following on from a lot of callous baiting, I was being pursued by an elder Dickensian-type pupil called Albert Kearns. Now if Albert had caught me, he'd have murdered me, that's no lie, but I'd sooner have suffered the death than be kissed by him because to me he was pretty gruesome (no offence, Albert)! Keeping this tale short, at one point whilst fleeing the irate Albert, I ran into Wansbeck dormitory. As I sprinted down the middle aisle between the two rows of beds, my attention was immediately focused on the tiny black and white television that sat in a corner on a raised shelf. Grandstand was on that afternoon and there was a running race taking place. As I skidded on the 3" thick shiny vinyl, I came to a temporary stop. I stood still, chest heaving, and briefly viewed a race from London's White City stadium while repeatedly checking over my shoulder. It was then that a name rang out with words to the effect of **'and the Morpeth man, Jim Alder, has taken on the pace'!** Surely I'd misheard – can't be right, a Morpeth athlete in London (where's that?), winning a race? There was little chance to take it in though, because Kearns reappeared at the bottom door, screamed an obscenity my way, and with no time to deliberate, I was off out the top door while doing my utmost to stay alive! *The right place right time* phenomena (clearly without me knowing) had occurred for me without any warning, and of all places in a wooden shed of a school called Brown Rigg Boarding School! Now that fiery sequence of events would mean absolutely nothing to anyone, but me, but was probably the onset (although I didn't know it then) of so many of my future athletic ambitions.

To: Jim Alder, Commonwealth Games Marathon Champion, we were always ships in the night, Jim, as would always be the case, regardless, for me you are an icon, in a blink of an eye, you'd replaced Nurmi, Zatopek, Bannister, Pirie and several others, and it all began for me in Wansbeck Dormitory sometime during the hot summer of 1965! You're still coaching, Jim, and in between bending in the street to pick up discarded litter, a long way from Olympic Stadiums. Wonder if Albert is still looking? – just as well that I now live in Chicago, Mozambique, and sometimes when I can be bothered Sydney?!! That's a long way from Berwick, Albert eh, not worth the airfare, my son, I hope!

There aren't many physical pursuits I haven't at least tried; some, it has to be said, are expensive and the better you get at the activity, well, the more expensive it all becomes and you need a never-ending cash outlay, either to initially purchase your equipment, or then to refurbish it as usage takes its toll. In contrast, walking, jogging, and running are perhaps the cheapest of all pursuits, as cheap as chips. Two pairs of trainers are better than one as they allow you to alternate them in terms of usage, thereby leading to a greater degree of longevity. There are literally countless makes; the best bet is to decide to what extent you want to engage yourself in the activity, i.e. twice a week, four times a week etc. Then I'd pay a visit to one of the specialist shops, tell the shop assistant how much you want to spend and what your aim is; it couldn't be simpler, i.e. you may be happy simply doing Park Runs or may want to progress up to a 10k, maybe leading up to a half marathon or whatever, distances and terrain clearly play a role in your choice of shoe.

Worried about how you look? Trust me, you aren't alone, MOST PEOPLE have reservations about their physical appearance, it's natural, but if you need it, you should get some 'comfort' from a basic fact – you are special, you are unique, and WE ARE ALL SO DIFFERENT! As we are all different, it makes sense to accept that we will all run differently.

A while back I watched an hour-long programme on the television about health and fitness. In my opinion the programme was aimed at all the wrong people, i.e. slim athletic types who are already partaking in exercise, but the larger market is the millions of people waiting to be 'coaxed' into the joy of 'basic' exercise. At various times during the programme the presenter visited several specialist venues and introduced us to another 'expert' who would explain in Greek what this, that, or the other, would do for us. At some point in the presentation, the viewer was introduced to an international athlete who was asked to demonstrate 'how we should run'. As the lithe super runner then gave an example on running form, i.e. in their opinion landing on the ball of your foot before pushing off from your toes to extend and increase your stride length, whilst keeping your upper torso upright additionally using your arms and shoulders to maintain form and drive. Go on, try it – if you're caught you'll get sectioned, that is if the officer can stop laughing long enough to retain you!

Does running style matter? Of course not! Here's a little story.

In 1948 the Olympic Games were held in London, the first games after the war, Wembley Stadium was full to the rafters and the first event was the men's 10,000 metres. With a crack from the gun off went the 30-plus athletes. A group of 'spectators' sitting in the stands got their eyes on a lowly figure wearing the red vest of his nation, who fell immediately to the back of a long drawn out orderly line. The athlete's face was already contorted in apparent agony as he attempted to 'hang on' to this elite body of athletes. The athlete's upper body rolled and rocked back and forward with exaggerated movements befitting 'exhaustion' – the field had barely covered one of the 28 laps! As this bunch of spectators continued to laugh and make fun, one of them shouted 'ha ha, look at him, he runs like us' as the runner continued around the track oblivious of everything apart from his supreme efforts! A short while later, the red vest was seen to slowly creep up through the straight echelon till eventually he was in the lead; his style if anything had further deteriorated. As the other athletes fell off the pace, the red-vested runner pumped his arms yet higher across his chest as his legs found even more energy. The group of spectators were no longer laughing! The athlete won by a considerable margin with a sprint finish as the spectators reached for their programmes to identify the best runner in the world, with the worst running style in the world. The red-vested runner was **EMIL ZATOPEK** *of Czechoslovakia! Over the coming decade, Emil went on to win another medal, silver, in the same London games in the 5k. Four years later in the following Olympic Games in Helsinki, he won an unprecedented three gold medals, in the 5,000, the 10,000 and then the Marathon, all in the same games and all with the style from hell! More world records and a further glut of European medals followed.*

My intention when writing a lot of this book, is once again to <u>'buck trends'</u>. I've been around the athletic world a long time, I've always been self-coached and I really don't need to follow others just for the sake of it, although I respect their views, of course! Now those ever-changing trends seem to come from the multiplying numbers of 'experts', many of whom are not athletic practitioners, and their continuous and never ending 'studies and research' are apparently handed down to them from professors, scientists and doctors who seem intent on turning a relatively simple subject (i.e. how to be healthy and improve or maintain your physical fitness), into a never-ending, complex and difficult to understand science.

(Talking of bucking trends, here is one I'd like to buck, and comes from yet another magazine article I've just read about 'training your brain'. Xxxxx (the author) can help you identify your feelings and to understand that they are our mental health muscles. Check in with your emotions, e.g. fear, guilt, shame, to discover what they are trying to tell you what to do next? Apparently, the author is a 'radical self-care advocate' and a psychotherapist and mental health consultant! My first thought is can you really make a sustained living out of the latter 'tip of the iceberg' confusing subject? Bet the celebs and stars are just drooling at their mouths!

In contrast to the above, running is a very simple activity – unlike cooking, for example, where there are literally thousands of different recipes, made possible by countless available ingredients. But running is so much simpler – and it's simpler by virtue of the fact that there are very few ways of running; I mean, the activity is not at all like complex dance routines or numerous gymnastic permutations. With running you are a single entity, it's just you and me, we don't operate with another in tandem and we don't mimic or replicate the same often complex movements, in fact all the runner does is systematically place one foot in front of the other at varying speeds. So, once we've initially mastered that 'instinctive' running action (and for most of us we master it from cradle to pavement in around four-six months), and after that brief learning curve, we never quite forget how it goes. So, adding to that basic non-complex philosophy, the runner's options are: we can run slowly, or at a medium pace or we can run fast (everything is relative, one person's sprint is another's jog). Additionally, we can run short distances, medium distances or long and even ultra-distances, and we can alter the terrain we run on!! End of! Despite the thousands of books all saying pretty much the same thing, running is not a complex art (remember, people make lots of money by convincing the rest of us they have some sort of special mystical knowledge, maybe derived straight from the Lab? And wouldn't we be foolish not to want it? After all, the source of the continuing 'new' info is from educated people with labels attached to them. Even if there is a monetary price to pay.

Come on, Micky baby, there has to be more to it than that! Otherwise, why are there coaches? Well the coaches, all of whom I have unreserved respect for, take the basic action of running and they carefully combine the activity with those commodities mentioned previously, that's pace, distance and terrain, blend those in with the ingredients of established running methods such as Intervals, Repetitions, Fartlek, Long Slow Distance (LSD) and with a bit of luck, the individual becomes a quicker and stronger runner. IN CONTRAST, WHAT IS AN ART (AND FEW ACHIEVE IT), IS TAKING ALL THAT AND HAVING IT COME TO FRUITION AT A PRECISE MOMENT IN TIME – AND THAT'S KNOWN AS THE OFTEN MYSTERIOUS ART OF PEAKING!!! BUT I'LL SAY IT AGAIN, RUNNING, A BIT LIKE CYCLING, IS PRETTY SIMPLE! Field events aren't, swimming isn't, gymnastics and table tennis aren't – but running is walking at pace, as such for the athlete, it has just got to make sense!

Let's go back to the programme mentioned above, and now ask yourself how many people on god's earth can run comfortably like the demo given by the elite athlete in the programme? Furthermore, ask yourself how the so called knowledgeable 'experts' could even contemplate the use of such a demonstration intended to make us all look pretty whilst ignoring the would-be athlete's 'instinctive action' – the programme was so far away from 'reality' it was almost farcical. Wonder whether the hosts had ever even heard of Emil?

My view, and again it doesn't make me right, is that we run the way we do because we find it most natural and most comfortable – if there was a better way then instinct would find it for us. It is quite well known that 'motor skills' (movement) are best learned, technique-wise, from a very early age, somewhere between the ages of 6 to 11, or thereabouts. With the latter, I'm talking 'feel' for the water when learning the various swimming disciplines, or perhaps gymnastic activities, ball control etc. Once we get over that youthful phase, our ability to learn complex motor skills deteriorates. There are numerous elite athletes, particularly those in involved in endurance-type running, whose leg running action is by no means text-book, even ugly but so effective. Emil Zatopek, and Vladimir Kuts after him, being just two. On the contrary, it is possible to alter your upper-body running action, that's much easier, enabling a degree of relaxation whilst conserving energy. Running can be a beautiful art form – watch Coe, Ovett or Cram, or Dina Asher Smith, but they're especially gifted! Zatopek once said 'track and field' is not like ice skating, you don't have to smile to influence the Judges. Indeed, it is difficult to smile at a camera when running!

Relaxation while running!

Everything in and on the body is connected to another body part, nothing works in isolation. As such, movement of one body part affects the movement of another. When you're running – relaxing your legs is especially difficult because they are working so hard; however, relaxing the upper body is much easier and a relaxed upper body (waist upwards) will save energy. Roll up your shirt and try this: make a fist, you can immediately see the effect the hand/finger has on your forearm – the tensed forearm now affects the bicep and the bicep is the instigator for tension in the deltoid (shoulder) and it all began with the fingers! If you want to relax the upper body while running, make a light cupping action with the fingers (not a fist) and try lowering your arms to a position a little way above waist height – the higher you raise your arms the more tension you will create. For most of my sporting life, I have complemented my cardio and legs with upper body strength work, press ups, dips, curls and shoulder press; and to do all of those you need nothing other than a chair and a pair of dumbbells. In summary, upper body strength can invariably improve your running action.

If you want to improve your stamina, then aerobic conditioning is appropriate – the longevity of the exercise helps create a bigger, stronger heart, lungs and oxygen transport system. Remember the heart is a muscular pump, and like all muscles if you carefully (gradually) exercise it through physical activity it will get larger and more efficient. The more efficient it all gets, the less the limitations will be. One of my oft used sayings is YOU CAN'T FAKE STAMINA, and aerobic activity helps create increases in stamina/endurance.

How about a combination of walking and running? Any pace or distance you like!

HERE'S AN IDEA STRAIGHT FROM THE ROYAL MARINE COMMANDOS

When I was a serving Royal Marine, we regularly performed a group exercise referred to as **SPEED MARCHES!** The idea of 'speed marches' was to cover a predetermined distance as quickly and as efficiently as possible, whilst remaining in a group; the aim was to reach the destination as a complete body of fighting soldiers whilst conserving enough energy and strength to allow us to perform a variety of military duties befitting Great Britain's elite fighting force. Stay with me, whilst I explain!

Speed marches are an 'ideal' method of incorporating aerobic fitness into your training week; furthermore, these are FREE, you don't have to do them in a group, and you don't need any expensive training equipment or a special environment, all you need is some recreation/sporting clothing and some appropriate footwear. Here's how they work.

Here is an example (the distances or times I'm using are simply 'examples', they aren't carved in tablets of stone, and there are numerous permutations you can use); you begin by starting your stopwatch or having a pre-determined distance you intend covering, and you're walking quickly (not flat out) for a period of time, i.e. one minute to five minutes, then you jog for one-two minutes, then slow down to another spell of fast walking for one-five minutes, follow that up with another even paced jog for one-three minutes, then you walk again, and so on and so on! Already you can see it's a terrific way of being outside in the fresh air (the beach? the park? football field, pathways or quiet roads, national park areas, or even a housing estate (if you're 'thick skinned' and like a laugh, ha!) whilst performing an incredibly effective way of aerobic (not totally out of breath) activity. Do it alone? Do it in pairs, do it with your kids or mates *'and if you ain't got any, do it with ya dog or ya orrible little moggie or 'even' your partner (yes I'm serious)*.

At a glance you can see the possibilities; you can do one mile or three miles, you can do two hours, or 20 miles, it's your shout; additionally you don't have to shoot people at the end, a bonus, for some! Any runners reading this will say 'that's fartlek that' (a runner's form of training) and you're right, only there is more discipline required with this one otherwise you'll end up operating too slowly or too casually, and as such the effect will be marginal.

I rate the above form of exercise so highly that I intend to do the very same when I get old!

SWIMMING

(a great exercise but you require time and the discipline of a working Monk!)

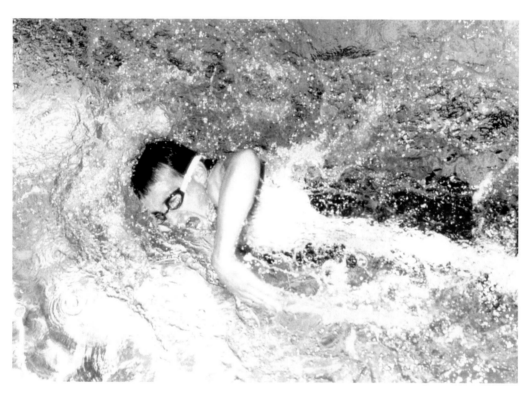

My introduction to swimming came when I would be around nine years of age, 1959-ish. The nearest swimming baths for me at Widdrington were about seven miles from home, so a visit, no money, no car, was absolutely out of the question, until that is when my mate Trevor Barnes mentioned one day during the long school summer holidays that his dad was taking him and his brother David swimming the following day and he'd ask his dad if I could go. Now, Jimmy Barnes (Trev's dad) had a 'mushy pea-green' coloured little car with an L sign prominently displayed on the vehicle's 'inside'; nevertheless the sign was clearly displayed, if only to show the terrified 'internal' passengers that he hadn't progressed far in the past 20-year learning period, whilst hiding his obvious inefficiency to the world outside. Anyhow, Trevor's enquiry got a 'yes no problem' reply, and fortunately my mother also agreed to this initial swimming debut, more so as there was no bus fare to find – I couldn't wait, my excitement was immense! The next morning my mother left for work shortly after 6am and as soon as I heard the door close downstairs, I was up and dressed, ready to go for an 8.30 departure and a place in the 9am early morning session. I lay on the settee for the next two hours silently watching the clock (hard to believe now, but there was no morning television in those days), and at 8.30 I knocked on Trevor's door and away the four of us went to Ashington baths. To this day I can recall the adrenalin deriving from the smell of the chlorinated water and the kids shouting and their shouts echoing off the tiled walls. None of us could swim (there was no school lessons in those days), so we just pretended with a variety of childish exercises as our toes barely reached the tiled floor in the 3'6" shallow end. The deep end in the 25yard pool was only 5'9" yet it had a spring board, a 'shoot' and a high dive and we'd regularly hold on to the side, kick our legs while watching the 'big lads' do their unsupervised pranks at the other end. What a day, truly wonderful, but there was to be no continuity until a year or so later, when I was allowed to go on the bus with my mates. We all got the exact money – bus fare there and back, and entrance money. After an hour in the water (where I was soon swimming up to 22 lengths!) we'd leave absolutely starving, hastily spend our bus fare home in Badiali's Café on the main street, before walking the seven miles home with an optimistic thumb in the air. Apart from an occasional visit to the baths when money could be found, the remainder of my apprenticeship as a swimmer took place at either Ulgham Burn or the beach at Druridge Bay. Who would have thought that in that very same pool many years later I'd spend a colossal amount of time going up and down whilst preparing to win British Championships! As well as teaching kids and adults how to swim properly as a qualified ASA Swimming teacher while being employed by Wansbeck District Council.

After my sparse swimming introduction at Ashington, and then throughout my military service where I always competed in swimming galas, as well as swimming for enjoyment, which occasionally entailed swimming from an anchored ship in some far-off tropical ocean. As mentioned later, I swam daily for many years, simply because I couldn't ignore it; it was a major part of my chosen sporting event – Triathlon. As a physical activity swimming has few rivals. It is a great all-rounder, few sporting pursuits can compare, more so because there are almost no, if any, injury-related problems, mainly because it is non-weight bearing, and as such it is very kind to the human form. However, for me personally, it ended there; I did it because I couldn't ignore it; it was an inescapable part of my competitive sport and therefore my life. But I personally found the onerous task of going up and down the pool every day of my life with nothing to look at but broken tiles for hours, almost soul destroying, which is probably why notoriously, competitive swimmers have limited competitive years, many swimmers are finished serious competition by their early twenties. It must be pointed out though that there are countless ways of bringing variety to your swimming work-out. There are the four main strokes as a starter, you can also incorporate intervals, time trials, repetitions and out of the water there are plenty of strength and conditioning activities to consider to add strength to the big muscles of the back (the Lats), the chest (pectorals), the shoulders (deltoids)and the triceps being the main movers. For the ordinary punter who has little in the way of competitive ambitions, swimming is also great as part of a 'cross training' programme once or twice a week, super as an alternative to running when injured, or as an 'active recovery' session. But you need time; additionally travelling to pools is also a thankless time-consuming task. I was so lucky during my triathlon years, I worked with a swimming pool at the end of the corridor (I even had access on Christmas Day and I used it) and when I 'unfortunately' got promotion to Assistant Manager and was forced to move to another location, I still had free access at the 'sister' site, but I rarely travelled with a smile. Outdoor swimming was in some ways more attractive and interesting, although the cold, even in a wetsuit was, well – it was – bah!!!

I never had a swimming lesson in my life, and learned to swim on rare visits to Ashington baths during the summer holidays, but it was fun, especially for a kid with a mountain of energy to burn!

To Barry Taylor and his very professional team of volunteers! There would be a huge gap without you all, Barry, you can't compete without competitive events and you put on superbly organised competitions. On hindsight the athletes have the easy job. In a culture whereby people can be quick to criticise and ever so slow to praise, on behalf of the thousands who have reaped the rewards of your efforts – 'our' grateful thanks!

Retaining your swimming form without going into the water! Following on from the Duathlon I did on the 23rd May 2021, I decided I'd do an 'Aqua/Bike' race (swim/bike – with a dodgy Achilles injury, no running was required) scheduled for the 10th July at the QEII lake, consisting of a 1,500 metre lake swim followed by a 46km bike section – the problem was due to the ongoing Covid virus issue as well as a bit of apathy, I hadn't swam at all since my last triathlon on the 19th August 2017, the latter incorporating a sea swim in the grimy North Sea at Sunderland! This event, somewhat misleadingly was referred to as the Sun City Triathlon – and it poured down!! Anyhow, with a little over five weeks to go to the QEII event and with some haste I went back into the lake at Druridge Bay Country Park and immediately swam, stress free for 30 minutes and found it an absolute doddle and invariably could have gone on indefinitely. Now in terms of triathlon, swimming was my weakest event of the three disciplines, so the question is *'how was I able to carry on swimming 'almost' where I left off three years ago'?* On reflection the only answer I can come up with is that, several days a week (more of a habit than anything) when I get off my bike or finish a run I always do bar-press-ups, dips, curls, shoulder press, abdominal work, core and stretching, the exercises were chosen for simplicity and all complement the muscular areas involved in swimming front crawl. Combine the latter with aerobic and anaerobic work (bike/running) and a feel for the water 'apparently' returns far quicker! No test tubes needed, just a bit of logic!

To Mark Breeze. I have always put too much effort into my cycling to potentially to get the bike mechanics wrong on race day! I am always grateful, Mark; your expertise has potentially taken away any unnecessary stress due to my personal inadequate DIY cycling maintenance! Forever grateful, Mark, many thanks.

CYCLING

(Still on the theme of aerobic activity, cycling is a magical exercise to enhance 'longevity' becasue it is non weight-bearing).

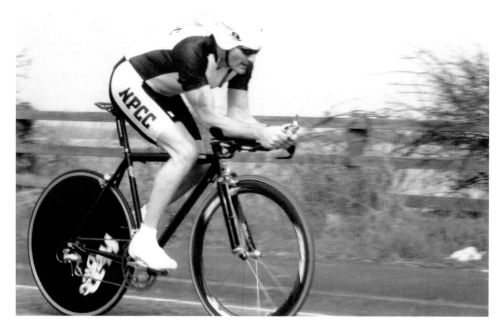

It doesn't have to hurt like this, I'm just short of recreational photographs!

But before talking cycling, give me a minute of your time – excuse the pun!

Computers and gadgets! – I well remember several years ago on conclusion of a 10-mile Cycling Time Trial event, and as the field stood ogling and analysing the result board, I approached an up and coming young cyclist and enquired how his ride had gone. He replied, 'Oh I was going so well, felt great, then I looked at my computer, and my heart rate was 'too high' so I backed off in regards to effort!' As he looked at the results of other riders he became somewhat subdued. It was a fast day and they don't come regularly, the wind was light, the traffic was kind, and several PBs were posted. 'Why did you back-off?' I said. He replied, 'My heart rate wasn't where it should have been.' Now in Time Trialling, the best riders go sub-22 minutes for 10 miles, and the exceptional riders go 20 minutes and under. I replied, 'You've missed a personal best time because of numbers on your computer!' He looked at me but was unable to respond, so to help him out I said, 'The whole event for you, is over in just 22 minutes and you backed off; if you continue to ride on those terms you'll never progress.' I then suggested, that for 10 and even 25 miles (the latter for faster riders is way less than an hour), your computer is a 'distraction' and you can do without it; however for 50 miles and 100 miles the computer becomes more useful on the grounds that it can keep you sensible in terms of riding the miles 'economically' and in a steady state so you don't jettison all your 'fuel' too early, nor do you want to shred your muscle fibres before the final 10 miles, and bonk. 'Bonking' and 'Hitting the Wall' are terms used to identify riding and running on 'empty' – OH HOW UNCOMFORTABLE THAT NIGHTMARE IS, AND THERE'S NOWT YOU CAN DO ABOUT IT, YOU'VE SPENT EVERYTHING YOU HAD AND TOO EARLY.

Sports Watches and Handle Bar Computers are now as common as sand at the beach, and millions of people spend their lives totally obsessed by the ever flowing data ('oops, what's wrong with me, my pulse rate is up 10bpm – help I must be dying!') and the data of course fluctuates continually during the course of a day as situations change (work, play, rest, temperature and 'mind games' as well as physical performances). The information, of course, is interesting and can be very productive; *however, the gadgets don't always tell you what you'd like to see!! I've always made a point in telling my small team of athletes, 'in the last 24 hours before your big event, turn the watch off, don't weigh yourself, and don't change a well-rehearsed routine, because you don't want any potential negative baggage, and the data is at this stage much too late anyhow. If you aren't fit on a Friday, you won't be fit on Saturday either.* Personally, I use one of the cheaper Garmin models occasionally, because it tells me, accurately, how far I've gone and how long it took me to do it. I have little faith in the heart rate info because mine fluctuates too much and to 'extremes'. I never use one on race days, my theory is simple – 'if I'm ogling my wrist or handle-bars every few seconds when racing at my max' whatever it's telling me, good or bad – truly doesn't matter!!

Tri-bars, here's a first – the first owner of tri-bars in the UK – and based here in 'little old' Widdrington in the midst of rural Northumberland amongst the pits and the farms. Who would have thought it!

In the 1980s I was sponsored by amongst others, a massive innovative cycling mail order catalogue based in London called Freewheel; all my bikes and additional cycling kit came from them. As such I'd travelled down to the smoke to do a photo shoot etc, pick up what I could carry, sign an annual contract and return home. Anyhow at some point around the 1980s, a suspicious package arrived at my door one fine day, and inside was an item I failed to make sense of. The item was a one piece lightweight metal 'object' with protruding sticky out tubes! Later I rang Freewheel and sought an explanation. During the chat they said they were the bees-knees and all the rage with the Californian triathletes (the nerve centre of world triathlon at that time), they told me to take them to Steels Cycle shop in Gosforth and get them attached to my bike. I knew the crew at Steels (the biggest cycling shop in the North East at that time) and it's fair to say there was some merriment regarding this new 'product' which I carefully placed on their counter – 'what are you going to do with those, Mike, ha ha, you'll be all over the road, man, no way can you steer your bike with those attached, you'll not be able to reach your brakes, it's a practical joke, are they taking the p..s? You'll be all crunched up and unable to breathe properly!' Anyhow to cut the story short, within a week or two 'everybody' was after these tri-bars especially having recently witnessed Greg LeMond win the final time trial stage of the Tour de France with another version of the bars secured to his low profile bike, in the process defeating the long term leader Laurent Fignon by a handful of seconds while taking ownership of the coveted Yellow Jersey. My usage of them was short-lived though, because the British Triathlon Association were quick to ban them on the basis that they provided an unfair streamlining advantage over the standard handlebars, and just like wetsuits at this time in the triathlon world, were not allowed in triathlon competitions!

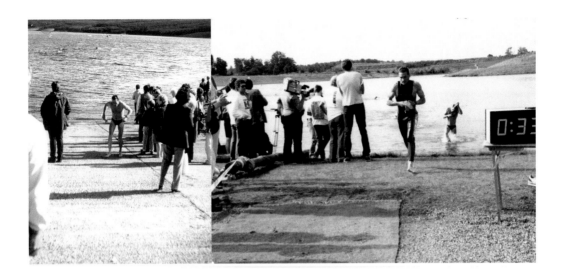

1983   *1992*

Wet suits were banned for a few of the early years!
Self-help only, being the philosophy.

*Hard to imagine now but for the first three or four years within the sport of triathlon **Wetsuits** were also a 'no no' as 'self-help' was the governance of the day and a strict criteria which ruled the world of triathlon (with a wonderful philosophy but one which wouldn't stand in the way of progress for too long), so freezing cold swims in trunks were the strict order of the day and all waterways such as the North Sea, rivers, lakes, reservoirs, ponds, puddles and quarries around the UK! **That's when men were men and had no willies for a week after a triathlon event (great for birth control) – they don't know they're born!**

I recall acclimatizing to cold water swimming by 'bathing' in the cold local QEII lake in March wearing trunks'!! where I got bitten and had the marks to prove it. A local fisherman told me without any sympathy ' that'll be a Pike, mate'! Madness is a virtue!

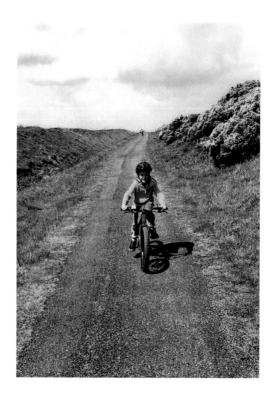

Very similar, Dan's first bike

My first bike!

Another of my childhood memories is from around 1960 when I would be *eight or nine years of age*, my dad had left home by then, and I'd persuaded my financially struggling mother to somehow buy me a bike. Anyhow, a short while later I excitedly accompanied Mother on the bus to Main's Cycle Shop on Ashington's Station Road to look at some bikes. I'd had a bike before, but it was a queer little thing with wobbly wheels and a bell that didn't work, and this mouth-watering possibility was the purchase of a brand new shiny one, maybe even with a working bell – can you imagine? I'm getting excited again at the thought. Anyhow, when we entered the shop, my mother, clearly with an eye on the cost, pointed at a couple of boys' bikes displaying prices, which clearly were within her shallow budget, and within a couple of seconds and an excited smile and a pointed finger I said 'I'll have that one please'. She agreed the terms of hire purchase, and as the HP details were being sorted out, I remember quietly asking if I could ride it home to Widdrington (about seven miles), which got an immediate 'don't be silly' reply! Once terms were agreed the manager added somewhat belatedly that there was a delivery fee, which clearly took my mother by surprise and her 'precise' budget was now somewhat lacking the additional delivery fee. Like a shot I repeated my earlier suggestion, 'I'll just ride it home, Mam', at which point my earlier 'silly suggestion' became an immediate 'good idea' suggestion and within 10 minutes, having had the seat lowered, I stood on the kerb on Station Road with the world's biggest smile and off I went as Mam went for the bus. *My 'first' bike race was on* as I attempted to ride the seven miles home before the bus got there. Anyhow, by the time Mother showed up, I was sitting on our back door step lovingly polishing the wheels.

Living rurally without cars, bikes were a wonderful, quick way of getting to the beach at Druridge Bay or up to Ulgham Burn, or going further afield gathering rosehips and conkers; most of those journeys would be accompanied by a passenger on the crossbar. I can even recall cycling with Alan Morton (he had three gears on his bike befitting his dad's wage as a Deputy at the pit) as far afield as Bamburgh and Tynemouth. At other times we raced around the blocks or even did 'time trials' to the 'old man's seat' at Ulgham and back; we didn't have watches in those days so someone sat on a kerb while quietly muttering – one elephant, two elephants, three elephants etc (with each elephant replicating a timed 'second') as you'd sprint around the final corner into the street and the last 50 yard sprint to the line you'd hear your time ringing out – 825 elephants, 826 elephants, you're three elephants slower than Trevor!!!

Fast forward 21 years and along came *Triathlon,* at which point I began racing bikes again, still without a bell, but with a proper stopwatch instead of the unreliable 'elephants'! I bought my first triathlon bike once again at a shop in Ashington, but this time the quality was just a bit better, although on reflection it was way too big. Regardless, I knew no better and rode this 24"Motorbecane bike (I should have been riding a 21 and half inch frame) for about two years, before I switched on and got a bike that suited my 5'8" frame. **40 YEARS LATER AND I'VE NEVER STOPPED RIDING – I'm talking bikes!**

I would state categorically and have absolutely no doubt whatsoever that riding and racing bikes has extended my active physical (or sporting) lifespan inordinately and enabled me to remain highly competitive right up to today, and today I've done a super cycling interval session. I can't think of another physical activity that gives so much more back without taking anything in return, except expense! Today (12/3/2021) and it's been a difficult ride due to very strong winds, I've rode again as normal for two hours, apart from some local muscular fatigue due to energy expenditure, I feel great, no aches, no activity-related pains, no stiffness... how can that be at 70 with a body that has truly been through the mill, that's following a lifetime immersed in extreme athletic pursuits? A current celebrity does adverts on the television because his knees hurt (ok, I know it's business) and here I am having done possibly more physical stuff than any athlete on god's earth and my knees are terrific as is my back, most of the time. Am I lucky? Of course, but have I made my own luck? Whatever, the bike has had a definitive positive effect on my athletic life.

Following the National Long Course Championships at Guernsey in 1993 when I was 43 (finishing 8th) I terminated my triathlon career; then at 50 years of age, after many years of competitive running, triathlon, swimming and ultra-fit competition, I returned once again to serious cycle racing (I needed something else in my life to challenge me). Following some real strenuous consistent training over the next 18 months I began to find winning form. I was 51 when I won my first open event and over the next decade I'd win more than 75 open time trials, in all sorts of distances, and all sorts of terrain and in all sorts of weather. NAME ANOTHER SPORT THAT WOULD ALLOW THOSE SORTS OF RESULTS AT THAT AGE? More to the point, name another sport whereby 'total' daily pursuit and flat-out physical effort allows you to beat people more than half your age whilst leaving no remnants of injury?

One of the great things about living in a semi-rural area, is that there are no boundaries such as traffic-laden roads or traffic lights to hinder your cycling efforts – put your shades and helmet on, then you wheel it out, climb on, clip in, set your watch and follow your nose for as long and with as much effort as you like – befitting your aim. If I were living in a city, things would be different but here it's sound.

Are there drawbacks with cycling? Yes, if you go looking for them. The weather can be hostile up here* if you let it get to you, there are many more riders out in the summer months than there are in winter (hibernation, it seems, is not just for squirrels and hedgehogs), bike parts can be expensive, (although I still ride winter bikes that I got in 1984 and 1985), drivers are occasionally out to kill (or so it seems) and positive physical feedback in terms of physiological improvement particularly on the cardio, are not (time out) as quick as the gains in some other physical pursuits such as running.

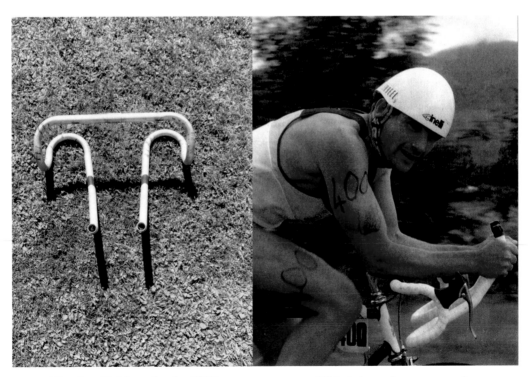

The first Tri-bars in the UK?   *This is how they were used*

RUNNING, SWIMMING and CYCLING!

(A comparison, I'll keep it brief)

Running is incredibly genuine and honest; wealth doesn't come into it, meaning you don't need anything expensive to run in, you need shoes and an array of simple clothing and off you trot. You can run almost anywhere (I've done it on roads, tracks, in woodlands and across farmers' fields, whilst standing in trenches with an 84mil' anti-tank gun for company, on ships as we rock and roll across the Bay of Biscay, then won a race up to top of the Rock of Gibraltar, in the heat of jungles as well as in the snowy Cheviots and on Dartmoor hills; I've ran in excessive heat as well as in the most hostile of snow storms while running 'on top' of hawthorn hedges. The cardio-vascular physical returns gained from running in terms of 'time-out' are far greater than bike riding – your heart rate is taxed more in running is what I mean, especially in shorter, faster runs – a 20-minute steady run can be a tester, depending on how you run it; 20 minutes steady on a bike can help clear your head after a drink, but physically your energy expenditure will be far less. Running is free from restraints such as traffic. BUT running is weight bearing, and as such, injuries are extremely common. Remember, unlike walking whereby there is always at least one foot on the floor, with running you have some of the time both feet in no man's land (in the air) and at other times whilst running you've at least one foot in the air and the 'plant' back onto the concrete can be hostile as can be the flight from take-off on the ground to air needed to propel yourself forward. As far as running-related injuries go, and I am relatively light on my feet, I have had occasional injuries from 13 years of age right up to my current 70 years. The older you are, the more hostile is running, although you can 'cut your cloth' to suit in terms of speed, surface and distance.

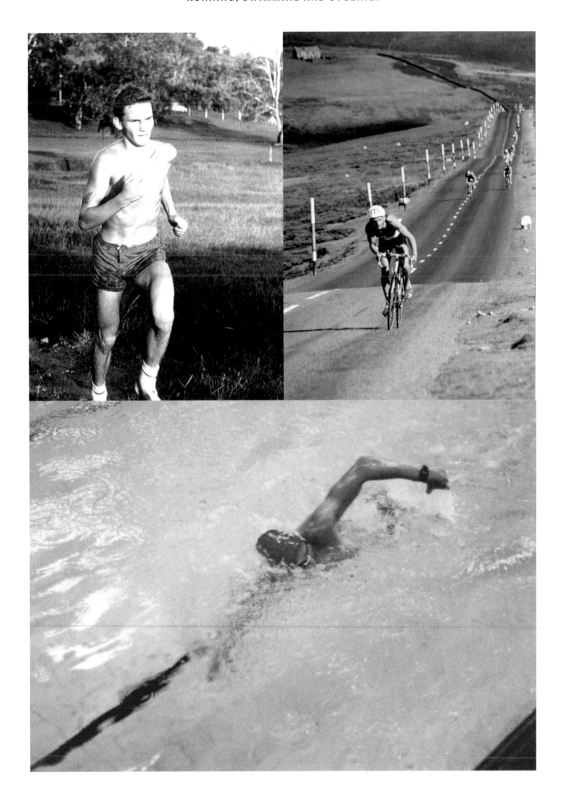

Swimming and 'pool exercises' are loaded with positives, the main ones are the friendly effect they have on the body, so picking up some sort of injury in a swimming pool is highly unlikely. Swimming works just about everything from the muscular side, except somewhat contradictable, little in the way of bone strengthening comes from non-weight bearing activities. Swimming is unlikely to strengthen or maintain bone strength, so we need some impact activities to develop, maintain, and improve bone strength. Having worked on pool sides it seems that what is instinctive is the magnet of hanging on to the pool side and kick our legs, few people remain 'still' in a swimming pool, rest periods are kept brief without even noticing because unlike some other activities, we are 'drawn' to movement in the water. Other benefits are that the swimming pool is socially friendly, and as such family-only sessions have been part of the programme for as long as I can remember. The only real downside with swimming 'indoors' is the time it takes to travel, queue-up, pay a monetary price, and get changed. As mentioned elsewhere, motivation is the devil in terms of exercise facilitation, we can 'always' find reasons for not working out and swimming (for the older person) is one of the hardest to arouse to form of enthusiasm – especially in winter, *and consistency in exercise is crucial.*

Cycling can be almost stress-free in terms of jarring, and because the legs circle smoothly it's non-weight bearing. I HAVE NEVER IN MY LIFE BEEN INJURED DUE TO RIDING A BIKE AND I'VE DONE UMPTEEN THOUSANDS OF MILES! Fast, slow, and with serious amounts of miles, but nothing in terms of injury. I have fallen off on rare occasions, of course, but that's different and not recommended. Biking can help to keep your lower body supple, and if you ride hills your upper torso can be tested as well as your legs as you use your arms, back, shoulders, as well as core. In terms of PAIN, cycling for me at least was never as 'severe' as running, even when I was trying to win and absolutely flat-out. In contrast the pain I tolerated in trying to win running races and triathlons was nothing but extreme. *Flat out running hurt everything,* and my cardio was screaming, of course it was – the effort which created the turmoil so it was my choice; with biking when working hard (unless you're doing intervals on a turbo – and that is similar to flat-out running) – well, sooner or later you will go downhill or have a tail wind so there is always some respite and recovery; also you have the bonus of changing positions on your bike, sitting or standing! Another consideration is the after-effect of cycling, maybe being a competent and everyday user of the bike helps, but the day following a hard biking session I am ready to go again, no ill effects. The opposite is true in relation to running, a hard run leaves me sore, more so with age and of course it is the repetitive jarring as the foot repeatedly hits the ground which is the culprit.

I once rode a 100-mile time trial on a 24" low profile bike at 6am, and finished a close 2nd. Went home had something to eat and ran 16 miles in the afternoon with Ben my springer 'setting the pace!'. I was training for an Ironman event at the time, but it seems the morning's efforts on the bike allowed the doubling up in the afternoon.

Running, Swimming and Cycling – a brief conclusion!

Incorporating the three activities into your athletic endeavours is a sound ambition, as the three are complementary to each other. When I am 'running seriously' I do more of it (running), I therefore use cycling as an active recovery exercise taking the emphasis from the rigours that come from a weight-bearing activity and putting it onto another non-weight-bearing activity. So, maybe I'll run five days in the week and cycle two. Cycling seven days a week is child's play – today is my 156th consecutive day riding a bike – amazing, all things considered!

I love the simplicity and the honesty of running. I despair at the amount of money my cycling rivals spend on 'better' equipment, and clearly if two people are the same in terms of ability and effort, the one with the better equipment will win (just like F1); in running little of that is an issue. Although as times move on, unfortunately, even running shoes are now being manufactured to offer the wealthier athlete a degree of one-upmanship. As far as I was concerned, I often lost out with kit, I had a family and money was always tight, I made do with what I had and what we (Jennifer and I) could afford. On analysis I always wondered how many events incorporating cycling I lost because my equipment was second best. When tests are done in wind tunnels, they tell you conclusively how much time you're losing because of what you're riding on and what you're wearing – well, you either smile and say 'well so be it' or you put yourself into debt and the latter wasn't something I could justify.

I've mentioned the principles of aerobic work before, so just a recap. Aerobic activity is steady state exercise, so after gradually elevating your pulse rate at the beginning of the exercise, you should then gradually take it up to around 120bpm to maybe 140bpm (that's a guide – bearing in mind that the 'resting' heart rate for an 'average' adult is around 70bpm). Once your heart rate has risen, the aim is to have it remain fairly consistent from that point onwards until you reach your pre-determined distance or time-out, the remainder of your intended workout remains 'aerobic', i.e. steady state rather than have it fluctuate. Your 'breathing rate' should act as a guide; you shouldn't be breathless – if your breathing becomes haggard, then slow down! Some use something called the 'talk test' meaning if you can converse with your training partner you aren't far away from where you want to be. Consistency is a huge requirement in stamina improvement, so if you want to identify improvement, do it regularly, a bare 'minimum' of twice a week, better still at three to four times. Bear in mind, we're all different, no two of us are identical, and I hope most of what I'm writing is a 'common sense' based guide. I regularly trained three times a day, seven days a week, but it was 'normal' for me, and you don't get to that level overnight, it's a long and gradual process, and as working 'amateurs' we all encounter many differing barriers. Now with barriers you either stop and go back, and take another easier route, or you do what I did, and you find a way to go over, under, or through them. Thank god many people are born wiser; and use the health benefits derived from exercise to enrich or enhance their lives; as such they have no desire to become a top athlete, and many top athletes are like me, boring, driven, and ever so selfish in our quest to be the best, but I'd hastily add, that doesn't make us better or even worse than anyone else, just a bit different maybe.

BEFORE MOVING ON TO *ANAEROBIC* ACTIVITIES, BE VERY CAREFUL ABOUT ALL THOSE ADVERTS!

Be careful! I wonder how many people over the recent couple of years have been 'injured' and forced to prematurely terminate their newly acquired enthusiasm for exercise due to jumping energetically around sitting rooms whilst trying to keep pace with the superbly fit host during video presentations and on-line presentations. I'm talking about people who have gone from sedately sitting and lying on the sofa to leaping around the lounge like there's no tomorrow. Short, sharp exercise can be totally self-defeating without some thought. Remember LONGIVITY is the name of the game!

BEFORE YOU BUY! CONSIDER THIS! Are you fed up with all the current every day repetitive adverts showing young 'attractive' (beauty as they say is in the eye of the beholder – so?) model athletes furiously working out on their expensive sitting room bikes with all the IT gimmicks that go with them? Well listen, it doesn't have to be that way. I can, with a degree of certainty, tell you that for the ordinary keep-fit person the 'short time' flat-out efforts associated with the big sell, and consequential long-time accrued debt, is almost deceitful. When you see the 'Adonis', or the 'goddess' that both models are so desperately trying to mimic, operating at 100 percent, legs spinning like the wheels of an F1 car, @ 500rpm, off their butt and out of the saddle, sweat cascading like rain during the monsoon season in the Malayan jungle, whilst saliva dribbles from their lipstick mouths off their chin and onto the elaborate Boeing 707 console, and yet despite the all-out effort the obligatory Colgate-white smile gets somehow wider, well, they are doing it all for money, sucked from your pocket like a powerful magnet and straight into theirs. Now who am I to offer caution? What I would say is simply this. **With exercise in general the biggest challenge for us all is <u>LONGIVITY</u>. Exercise that insists on, or is portrayed as 'flat-out' exercise, is rarely designed with the ordinary keep fit and health orientated enthusiast in mind; additionally the torment you encounter in flat out efforts will not be gleeful and unlike the models you won't be ecstatic at the thought of it as an everyday or even every**

other day health related panacea. **Categorically, there is little in the way of 'longevity' when administering self-inflicted PAIN. Pain can be a big de-motivator.** Within a week of the purchase many will wake up on day five and say 'oh god, no not today – please'! And god will reply 'ok, take a day or two or three off'. With that, the would-be sadist smiles, touches their toes, swings their arms, does a few sit-ups, and retreats to the sanctuary of the comforting daily pre-work shower.

The above discussion revolves around **anaerobic** exercise and anaerobic exercise is by definition 'hard' physical work, intended for the very fit, and how do you quantify the term and condition of the 'very fit'! **Here's a personal little secret, which I've never openly mentioned before. At my current age of 70, I have increasing personal reservations about hard anaerobic physical work-outs. It somehow doesn't currently seem sensible to thrash myself to extremes. My guide is this – would I recommend this type of exercise to other 'elderly' people? And my answer is NO! With the body (unlike lifting the bonnet of a car to look inside at the workings of the engine) you can't zip yourself open and peer inside, and 'intense' physical activity presents a risk, and not just from the increase in physical injury but also from the cardio perspective. If anaerobic exercise can be performed at 75 per cent effort, I'll work with that, if it means (as a 70 year old athlete) I must go to 95 percent of max, it ain't worth the risk; as such (although even today I've done a cycling interval session) there won't be any more for me at that intensity, whatever the risk is, it outweighs the benefit, such is age!**

As mentioned above, aerobic exercise is defined as 'with oxygen' and so anaerobic exercise is precisely the opposite – and is performed 'without oxygen', so the severity of the exercise creates major limitations. The limitations are brought about by insufficient time which is required to suck in enough air and to transport it to working areas of the body, ultimately to satisfy the body's demand. Anaerobic activities are at the hard end of exercise, 'athletes' who have designs on competitive ambitions normally incorporate between one and three weekly anaerobic training sessions within their measured training plans depending on how fit they are, and for many the day after the hard session is an easy recovery day. Now I'm not saying there is no place in the 'keep-fitter's' day for harder anaerobic training, because there are advantages to working harder on some days, what I am saying is that if you believe based on the current everyday adverts that every morning you are going to jump from your bed and leap onto the miracle bike for another beasting, well, you are kidding yourself.

For serious ambitious athletes, anaerobic training is essential, mainly because it mimics the pain and distress they encounter in competition; in other words it conditions the athlete, whilst also making physiological changes in the body. In competitions when all things are equal, i.e. pace and stamina, the real decider will be 'pain tolerance' – who can withstand the most pain and discomfort and still find the motivation to push on. During such times there are mind-games and athletes, of all specialist activities, are continually wondering about their opponents, are they hurting as much as you, or are they ready for the taking with one more surge? Here are a few chosen words on anaerobic exercise.

NEED SOME INSPIRATION?

THROUGHOUT THIS BOOK I HAVE TRIED IN MY OWN LITTLE WAY TO MOTIVATE PEOPLE TO LOOK AFTER OURSELVES, ALTHOUGH SOMEWHAT CONTRADICTABLY, I DO BELIEVE YOU HAVE THE ABSOLUTE RIGHT TO LIVE YOUR LIFE HOW YOU CHOOSE AND WHATEVER YOU DECIDE HAS LITTLE IF ANYTHING TO DO WITH ME. Nevertheless, **have a look at this please!**

David Grieves!

A short while ago I read a book called *Bubbles, Blood, Sweat and Beers* authored by my good friend Dave Langdown (drummer/publican/businessman/ entrepreneur), and the book was an excellent insight into another bloke's life, well away from athletics! Anyhow, one chapter within the book really touched a nerve and was called HEROES. Dave's hero in this instance wasn't a rock star, footballer, film star etc. His hero was in fact a local guy called *David Grieves.* Drenched in emotion, Dave went on to talk about David (whom I never knew), explaining he was born with a severe heart defect, as such was in and out of hospital all this life from infant and child to adult and beyond to his untimely death at 50 years of age in 2009. Clearly the latter medical condition (excuse my terminology) resulted in non-participation of so many activities, activities that most of us take for granted yet were inhibited or ruled out of David's life because of his condition. Now I have repeated many times how many of us, or perhaps most of us, don't realise what we've got till it's all too late and it's gone, basic health comes into this throwaway supreme asset, and once we've kicked it into touch, well, it's gone and try as you may we struggle to get it back, and in many cases it's gone for good! David never had what most of us had, simple good health, the greatest gift of all, he was dealt such a poor hand at birth, not his fault, but he managed his life as best he could and even worked for Dave, becoming a supervisor in one of his bars. David once quietly told Dave he had one major ambition, you know what it was? – ***"to run the full length of his street!"***

Now I am a sensitive soul, I can't help it! If you've read my other books you will have gathered how emotional I can be in respect of certain subjects, and the latter little story has left its mark!! As many of us sit around just too lazy to 'move', there are others who would give everything just to be able to participate, not to be good at it, or to win – just to be there and be part of it all and enjoy!

Wished I had known you, David Grieves – god bless!! And in the next life I wish you the best of everything!

ANAEROBIC ACTIVITY

A STATEMENT OF EFFORT IS A STATEMENT OF CHARACTER!

(I believe, on some occasions, you can learn more about a person's character in a gym or park run than you ever can by sitting them behind a desk and putting a pen in their hands.)

Contrary to popular belief, physical 'effort' is not dependent on physical prowess. Effort more than anything is an 'expression'; it relies little on skilled-based ability, and is honesty personified. An accompanying verbal statement would bluntly read 'this is what I'm about, take it or leave it' or 'what you see is what you get'! And I believe athleticism takes a back seat to the 'effort' given during many physical pursuits. Here's another thought: whilst there is normally only one outright winner, that doesn't mean all the others are losers, far from it; in every race or competition there can be hundreds of 'personal' races, and when you come out the other end you know whether you've been victorious; indeed if you couldn't have given more – you've won – terrific!! Sports of all varieties have one thing in common: they are character building. On the occasional events I've spectated, I could build 'my special army', not by choosing the victorious, rather by selecting the brave!

Ok, we know that aerobic exercise is steady state endurance activity; well, anaerobic exercise is quite the opposite. Anaerobic exercise is where the body's demand for oxygen is 'not' being met, and that's due to the severity of the work-rate. Anaerobic activity causes us to get quickly out of breath – that's referred to as creating 'oxygen debt' – and the debt we've built up during the exercise causes breathlessness and muscular fatigue which must be paid back and we pay it back by slowing the exercise rate down or stopping. The latter, of course, is not dissimilar to the monetary debt we can incur by reckless spending; in both cases if we spend too much of either oxygen or money then there is a debt to pay – in the first instance by slowing down or stopping the exercise till we recover, or in the second, talking nicely to the bank manager.

Typical anaerobic activities include: sprinting, cycling very hard up a steep hill, a competitive game of squash, lifting a maximum weight, flat-out swimming, and an energetic scrap in a street, as well as some forms of martial arts. The pulse rate during the above activities is very high and even maximal or approaching max!

The fittest man around is knackered inside a minute!! Many years ago, as a self-coached champion triathlete I used a system called 'periodisation' to get myself 'spot-on' and 'racing fit' at certain points of the year, i.e. to enable me to peak in a specific important race on a particular day of the year. I'll condense this rather than going into major and potentially boring detail.

So, I'd spend the winter months from December till the end of March building aerobic fitness, that is a huge engine capable of shifting countless gallons of oxygen carrying blood around my superbly fit body. Three times a day training was the order of the day: swimming before work, running during my lunch break, and cycling in some form after work, with a few weights thrown in when I could find both the time and the space. It was mainly steady miles, which you'll now recognise as aerobic training. Additionally, I'd occasionally attend Judo sessions at Ashington (I was a black belt in taiho-judsu – a combination of judo and aikido). Now considering the amount of physical training I was doing daily, you'd assume the judo sessions would be like taking candy from a baby, eh? They were in fact the hardest work-out of my very energetic week! Why? Simple! The Judo exercise was in total contrast to my aerobic sessions, Judo was in fact all about ANAEROBIC efforts, which as you now know were short, immensely demanding bouts of throwing, pulling, pushing, tripping, wrestling, and striking 'scraps'! Within seconds of standing on the mats I was drenched and my pulse rate (which at rest was often around 36/38bpm) would elevate up and over 180bpm, my body temperature would soar inducing copious amounts of sweat! Working so hard would ensure rest and recuperation was soon required, and yet at the time I was the best triathlete in the country (and

British Ironman record holder) – doesn't make sense, does it? Now had the judo taken place after April, when I'd be incorporating anaerobic work into my training – well, the judo would have been a lot easier for sure?

Successful athletes are successful because 'they do the right training at the right time'!

Back briefly to anaerobic training. Here's a 'simple' example of anaerobic work: 10-15 minute warm-up (jog, stretch, few faster strides and walk back) followed by 10x100yd sprints, pulse high, walk or jog back after each effort. Jog and walk cool down, stretch and shower!

Be careful with anaerobic training. Due to the severity of the work, which is normally with a heart rate 95% of max, the bodily stress encountered not just on the cardio-vascular system but also on muscles, tendons and ligaments is extreme, so the injury potential can be high. Purely as a general guide, anaerobic training even for the very fit should not exceed two sessions of the same activity twice within the same week. However, as a triathlete with three disciplines for consideration, there is more scope because of shifting the stress from swimming to cycling to running and back to swimming.

SO YOU CAN SEE WHY I AM A BIT SCATHING IN RELATION TO THE 'ADVERTS' COAXING ORDINARY PEOPLE INTO QUITE EXTREME PHYSICAL WORK-OUTS, IN BOTH CARDIO AND LIMB. THE CHOICE IS YOURS, OF COURSE, BUT BE CAREFUL!

ADDITIONALLY, I'M CONVINCED THE HIGH DROP OUT RATE ASSOCIATED WITH 'HERE TODAY, GONE TOMORROW' GYMNASIUM USERS (OR THOSE WORKING OUT ANAEROBICALLY IN SITTING ROOMS) IS CONTRIBUTABLE TO THE 'SEVERITY' OF THE EXERCISE THEY UNDERTAKE! WITH EXERCISE IN GENERAL, LOOK FOR 'LONGIVITY' – THAT'S 5 TO 10 TO 20 YEARS FROM NOW, I.E. A LONG TERM COMMITMENT. MY PERSONAL PHILOSOPHY IS SIMPLE: THERE IS NO POINT IN BEING FIT AND HEALTHY IN

YOUR 30s, 40s, 50s and 60s IF YOU ARE UNFIT IN YOUR 70s or even 80s. Take it easy today and you might just come back tomorrow; none of it should be designed to be a punishment!

Interval training, Repetition, Fartlek!
(I find myself writing much more than I intended)

I read an article a while back by a very well-known doctor, who suggested that a six-minute high intensity work-out was far better than a 30-minute easier physical session. Now there are pros and cons with just about everything; however, the suggested gains created through High Intensity Interval Training (HIIT) are that you'll gain a lot in a short time, heart, lungs and local muscular development. However, the risks involved in training in short flat-out terms are a real increase in potential injury, and if you're injured, well, it is clearly self-defeating. The 'unfit' person who is somehow enticed into the very hard short-term interval training work-out is taking a risk. Also as stated previously when you train hard you need longer recovery periods afterwards, whereas training easier allows more frequent sessions – 'you pays your money and …'

There are a lot of words of wisdom currently doing the rounds regarding High Intensity Interval Training (HIIT). The way it is currently portrayed suggests that this is a 'new' magical method of training – however, this type of training method been around for approximately 80 or 90 years, and was highlighted in the 1940s by a German athletic coach called Gerschler. His research was in-depth, and there was and indeed is a lot of supporting information regarding the positive effects of interval training. Emil Zatopek was its biggest exponent and he won three Olympic gold medals in the Helsinki games of 1952. However, he did his intervals at a lot slower rate than those advertised today. Zatopek did hours of intervals in one training session on the track, e.g. 20x200yds followed by up to 40x400yds and then finishing with 20x200yds – incredible! However, his efforts were often at race pace, then there was the recovery after each, so different from 'flat-out' efforts. So, with Zatopek he got race specific speed training whilst also gaining in stamina (because of how many he did) which enabled him to win from 5km right up to and including marathon.

Kids know what they're doing and they don't need computers or Fitbit watches – Watch and Learn!

I used to do all the above training methods as an eight year old (62 years ago), when I was playing in the dark winter months around Widdrington's challenging roads, garden paths and broken gates, privet hedges and iron railings, and short cuts, all of which were surrounded by the quiet car-free streets around our council houses. Of course, I didn't know it then by the terms of 'interval training or the current 'HIIT' or 'fartlek training' or 'repetition training' or even hill sprints, but our energy-sapping efforts had the same ingredients and the same benefits, as those performed with a coach and stopwatch on a measured 400 metre track. The missing link that changes the track training from the fun games was 'discipline'. We ran often flat out for lengthy periods till we either escaped our pursuers or we caved in and were caught. We'd run till exhausted while being chased by an opposing team member, then we'd instinctively rest, while being bent over double and inhaling and exhaling copious amounts of oxygen and carbon dioxide to and from our labouring lungs, then we'd do some more 'reps'.

It wasn't my intention when writing this book to write anything that had been written at length before, but when talking physical training that's impossible, so if there is replication, my apologies; however, when talking methods of training some are carved in tablets of stone, they work, when performed in the right manner. So in summarising differing types of quality training, we have:

Interval training: Can be performed over varying distances, the distances are often dictated by the specifics of a competition. So, it may be 10x 100m with a jog back recovery, or 10x400m with a 400m jog recovery, or 10 x 1 minute hard on a bike with one minute recovery spin, or even 10x75 metres in the water with 20 second recovery between each effort. There are countless permutations, you go hard for a time (at race pace or quicker), then you go easy to allow either partial or full recovery, then you repeat. The quantity is dictated by your aims and more so by your current fitness standard.

Repetition training: Is slightly different from interval training in so much as the efforts are longer and the recovery is longer and without the same intensity (possibly like those mentioned earlier that Zatopek was doing), so, the athlete may consider 4 x 800metres with five minutes recovery between efforts, the pace could be around race pace or slightly quicker; or 6 x 1000metres with six minutes recovery. When I was training for marathons, I used to do a two-mile warm-up, followed by 8 x 1mile at sub five-minute mile pace with a mile jog back as recovery, then a cool-down. In some respects, those sessions weren't a lot different from Zatopek's, at least in theory, except he was training towards 5 and 10km on a track, mine were on a measured stretch of quiet and mainly traffic-free road as per the marathons I was aiming for.

Fartlek training: could be described as a combination of the above, with less discipline where efforts or distances aren't carved in 'tablets of stone'. So, a brief example could be: 400 metre jog followed by 50 metre brisk followed by 100 metre steady then 200 metres 'quick' striding out, 200 metre jog and an 80 metre up-hill sprint with a recovery jog down etc. If you are working out in a group, each member can dictate the next effort; it keeps it all interesting and unpredictable depending on the pain inflicted on the members.

Endurance (over distance runs) runs: So, a 5km club athlete may contemplate doing a 10mile steady run as part of their weekly programme (Aerobic) as a means of increasing their stamina. As a 'guide', and there are exceptions, running twice or even thrice (depending on racing aspirations), their favoured race distance clearly the later example has the runner doing three times more miles than their racing distance which creates both stamina and confidence. A marathon runner may cover their long run of the week (or maybe every 10 days or so) as a 20-mile steady/easy run (aerobic).

ALL THE ABOVE QUALITY WORKOUTS CAN BE TRANSFERRED INTO THE WATER (clearly changing the distances) AS WELL AS ONTO THE BIKE (whilst increasing the distances!).

If you are interested and would like more info on the above training methods there is quite a lot of stuff in my second Autobiography 'Sixty years an athlete'(part two – filling in the gaps'). Available on Amazon.

Putting it all together and forming an appropriate personal training programme – here's a basic philosophical and much condensed guide – if you're a novice I hope it makes sense!

Deciding what you want to achieve means, perhaps above all, being realistic – don't copy intricacies from others, be brave and be your own person because as mentioned previously we are all in our own way unique with differing levels of available time, then there's our current physical standard to take into consideration, additionally there is next year's aims to consider in your forward progressive plan, the latter summed up as *short (this year's) and long term* (next year's) aims.

So setting out your Aims and Objectives (write them down in the front page of a training diary) keeps you on the desired straight and narrow achievable journey. Remember the reason for identifying 'aims' is to be logical and act as a pertinent guide as you move forward.

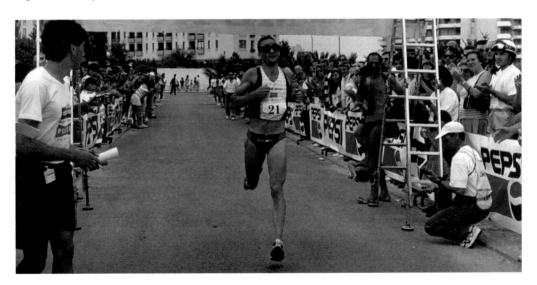

Sprinting, even after two hours of hectic activity, is necessary, which of course changes the activity from aerobic to anaerobic.

PARK RUNS

("You going for the win, Mick?")

On the 29th September 2014, I stood on the start line at Druridge Bay Country Park with so many other runners for my first ever 5km Park Run. With a couple of minutes before the off, I was approached by Stax (that's Dean Stackhouse, a mate of my son David's) – "You going for the win, Mick?" said Stax, accompanied by a confident nod of his ugly head. My anonymity sadly broken and nowhere to hide, I replied with an incredulous grin, "You must be joking!" At the time I was an inch away from being 64 years of age and on this chilly Geordie morning I was feeling every energetic year of it. My 'self-*talk' was anything but optimistic, as I* muttered to myself 'what the hell you doing here, Harris at 9 o'clock on a cold Saturday morning, you're the oldest person here, and you look it, you should be in bed, you dick!'

A few weeks earlier, having decided on a whim to return to triathlon, I'd had a few tentative training runs designed to complement my swimming and cycling, both of which were going well, but the runs were not as kind as the other two disciplines, and following such a lengthy lay-off I was already struggling with several running-related aches and minor injuries. So, this *was my first 'semi-competitive' run for about 20 years, having spent the last 15 years or so racing successfully on my bikes. Stax's comment had stirred me, though, and now there was nowhere to hide. I still had a mountain of personal pride regardless of age, and now his ridiculous comment had given me a boost of unwelcome adrenalin. I had been a quality athlete winning all sorts as a 'running races' but now instead of relaxing and basking in numerous memories I was about to subject myself to embarrassment and, who knows, even ridicule!*

A brief few words were given by a marshal before all too soon there was a countdown, 10, 9, 8... and we were off, habit had me standing close to the front and off we sprinted. 'Bear with it, Mick, it'll get easier, son' were my immediate somewhat comporting and repetitive thoughts. Needless to say, it didn't get easier and I laboured around the two laps, hurting and in a bit of oxygen debt. BUT I actually finished in 6th place, running 19m 51s! AND I WAS HOOKED. I travelled home, playing some Booker T and the MGs, had a bite to eat, took my bike out and rode for two hours. Once again, and 20 years since my last triathlon in the national long course championships in the distant Guernsey, I was excited and pleased to be a TRIATHLETE, albeit an old one!

To date, at February 2021, I've completed 57 events on various courses, I 'race' them all, flat-out, I give everything I'm capable of, every event, my mean average over the 57 events is 19m 47s (to get your past times you just click on your name and all your past results will appear, magic), my last 20 have all been sub-20 minutes and I'm a whisker from 70, and my first one almost six years ago was my most painful! Because of pride and the throw away comment from my friend Stax! (Thank you, mate!)

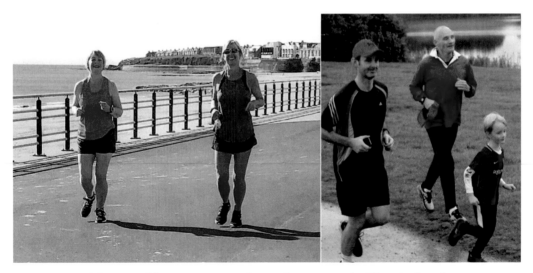

You are neither too old nor too young for park runs, as the Harris clan demonstrate. Clare and Lindsay 'brigten up the day' with their smiles.

PARK RUNS – ARE WONDERFUL!

The first thing I'd say, I hope reassuringly, is that park runs don't have to be competitive, nor do they need to hurt, they're called runs but you don't have to run all or even any of the 5km distance. There are thousands of events all over the world, they're free, you enter on-line and just turn up with your printed piece of personal data, cover the distance, hand your tag over to one of several marshals as you cross the finishing line, and your time will be recorded for you; it really is as simple as that! In my neck of the woods there are several events within a 15-mile radius of where I live, and I, like you, can turn up at any of them unannounced and take part. The organising marshals are remarkable, they are volunteers who turn-out every week, and are helpful and welcoming. The 'athletes' are warm, often humorous and full of banter defining the relaxed atmosphere. Some people are there to test themselves (club athletes), but many have no aspirations apart from covering the distance and getting their personal time, and once the event is over there is a very evident 'feel-good' factor as people, families, and mates enjoy the weekly gathering.

All the nationwide park runs begin at the same time every Saturday morning, that's 9 o'clock sharp, (once the Covid virus restrictions are lifted), but don't forget to take your printed tag with you otherwise you won't get your individual time and place, if indeed the latter are important to you. On conclusion of the event and depending on the venue you can have a post coffee, tea, or soft drink, and a chat to others or just return home to your bacon and eggs – till next week. I can't recommend these events enough, there're excellent! Numbers of participants vary from 50 or 60 to several hundred. In my experience, many people arrive too late – not to take part, rather too late to enable any last minute prep, such as a warm-up. Warm-ups for each of us are as different as chalk and cheese, but it's wise to walk around for 10 or 15 minutes, maybe partake in a bit of slow jogging followed by a few stretches. Jumping straight from your vehicle and sprinting to the start is not a great practice. There is also a 'safety briefing' lasting a few minutes, particularly aimed at people attending for the first time. There may be issues concerning the course as well, so best to attend.

PERSONAL BESTS (PBs)

Many people start Park Run events with the sole aim of *covering the distance* and that's great; however, once you've completed the distance, there is for many (not all) another almost immediate incentive which is to go quicker in the following events and surpass your last 'personal best' time. I'll state the obvious: *a 'personal best time' means you have today gone quicker than you've ever gone before in your entire life, and for anybody, that's just a bit special, an understatement!* Your time is almost silently stating, you've *never been this fit in your life* before – to date, bah!!! Nobody could make that happen for you, you've worked for it and you've reaped the reward of effort, so be proud!

Listen, let me add a few brief personal comments. In a race or Park Run there is nobody more important than you and your family (if your family is with you). OK, there is always a winner, the first across the line individual, and that being the case the 'winner' gets the adulation, the accolades, and perhaps a few pats on the back – job done; but I mean this most sincerely, the people at the back are probably more interesting than those at the front and that's because (just in my opinion, as I'm writing the book) the ones at the front are so immersed in their own selfish (no offence intended, I'm one of them) ambitions, but outside of their sport they may have little of interest to offer. Now in contrast, the people further back live in a wider world and keeping fit whilst covering 5km is a small but important part of their 'oh so busy lives', and the Saturday morning event adds immeasurably to who you/they are. I have lapped people in Park Runs, and some even step aside so I can get through, some even give me a shout – *'awesome'* one lady screamed – but your efforts are at least my and the winner's equal, that's for sure! Hope I don't sound stupid, regardless I mean every word.

To improve in anything there are tried and tested methods designed to help. If you always do what you've always done – you'll nearly always get the same end result. As an example: if you always run the same distance three times a week, at the same speed, then any overall improvement will be either unlikely or at best minimal. Now that's ok, of course, if your aim is to 'maintain' (rather than improve) your level of fitness. But if you decide you'd like to advance, add a spark to your efforts, then there are various well tried and tested ways of improving, in this case, your running 'times' or maybe increasing the 'distance' covered. The brief information that follows is designed with the 'casual' runner in mind (as opposed to the athlete – most of this book is not designed for 'athletes'), otherwise I'll saturate the next ten pages with just too much potentially confusing information accompanied by perplexing unnecessary textbook terminology.

This chapter is still largely about **'aerobic' activity** and walking, jogging and running are perhaps the easiest to participate in. I make that assumption not in relation to the physical sense, rather because you need nothing in terms of equipment to take part other than a pair of trainers – you can do the three activities in your pyjamas if you like, although some sports apparel will make your participation more comfortable.

In some respects what follows is folly and that's because (unlike those HIIT sessions portrayed on the television adverts) no one training programme can possibly fit all. I'll state the obvious: *we are all so very different; different aims, different abilities, different gender etc.* The examples of the four training weeks which follow are designed as a very simple guide, aimed at the 5km Park Run novice. So please be clever and take all of that into consideration. I'll give four possible training schedules which at least give an insight into what a balanced training programme looks like.

1. **A runner/walker with a 5km Personal best time of between 40-50 minutes.**

   Beginning on the **Saturday** with your **5km timed** run/walk.

   Sunday, 'Stamina' day: the aim is to build up time out or distance, so it's an aerobic session.

   1 hour speed march (see earlier chapter), walk and jog; Something like

the following: 5 minutes fast walk followed by 5 mins jog, 4 mins walk and 4 mins jog, 3mins walk and 3 mins jog, 2 mins walk and 2 mins jog, and repeat the sequence from 2 mins back up so you are finishing with a 5 minute walk and jog. So the session means you are on your feet for almost an hour.

Tuesday, Speed related, an interval session preferably on soft surface such as a football field. Warm-up is a 10mins walk and jog followed by 5 mins stretching. Followed by 10x50metres faster stride (half way line?) with a 50metre fast walk back to start, and repeat 10 times. Finish off with 10mins walk and jog cool down and some stretching.

Thursday, 2 mile jog! The aim is, or will be in time, to jog the 2 mile distance without walking, so initially as slow as you like but try to jog the entire 2 mile or the 20/25mins time out.

2. **A runner/walker with a 5km Park Run time of 30-40minutes.**

The above pattern can be used again, that's four times a week activity, fitted in around the Saturday Park Run. So, a longer session for stamina, a shorter session to incorporate a suitable anaerobic workout with 'intervals', a steady run to mimic park run conditions; remember to leave sufficient recovery gaps between training and the event, if you intend to try for a personal best.

3. **A runner with ambitions to go below 30 minutes for the 5km Park Run.**

OK, so you are looking more specifically at 'pace' now, and to run sub-30minutes if my maths is correct is around 9-minute miles. With the latter, conditioning the body to run at a specific speed comes about by subjecting the body to the aim. Your weekly programme can still entail four training runs. A longer session on the Sunday, anaerobic session on a Tuesday, but rather than 'intervals' I'd suggest 'repetitions' (review them above if you're still unsure how these work). Here is an example: warm-up jog and stretch, followed by 4x600metres at 9min mile pace or slightly quicker (or 4x800 metres). After each effort, you give yourself a full aerobic recovery period, e.g. walk around or jog 'very' slowly till your breathing rate returns to normal (don't allow your body temperature to drop too much) then you repeat the anticipated race pace repetition again. Once you've done your 2, 3, or 4 efforts, enjoy your cool-down and feel good, based on the reassuring – I can run 9min miles and that is around your current 30-minute aim.

<u>Note:</u> I'll say it again, don't let me pressurise you into something you aren't happy with. The advice is nothing but a 'possibility'; however, for some, being competitive maybe takes away the joy or personal satisfaction you currently get from 'comfortably' completing the activity, without being at all concerned about going quicker. BUT, if you feel you'd like to test yourself a little more then the above basic advice should provide some understandable guidance. This may strike a chord – if I had 10 park runners/walkers I'd probably offer 10 different programmes; however, as far as creating a balance goes, I'd still have (as above) four differing elements in the programme as follows – the actual weekly Park Run itself, one longer over distance endurance run (aerobic), one faster (anaerobic) and one steady run – that's four workouts in the week and three potential rest or active recovery days between them. One last thing: if your training/exercise remains static with no change, then your fitness will probably remain static and that's fine because you are maintaining your health. However, to see improvement, your exercise should be **progressive** (adding on more or going quicker). **Be specific** (table tennis will not make you a more efficient runner). And possibly above all, you should be **consistent**. (Whatever you do, do it all regularly.) As I said throughout this book **longevity** is the main aim.

This is really important. It is so very difficult for someone like me to write down an appropriate schedule, hells-bells I can't even see you, I don't know who you are, let alone prescribe something pertinent. Doctors are doing it now, sitting in offices prescribing medication without an on the shop floor office discussion, it's absurd! In all my life I've worked on the principle that if it makes sense, I'll try it, if I screw my face up and think – 'hell, that can't be right – can it?' I'll ditch it. Remember, running is simple so keep it that way. With all the above examples, the bright person 'selects' an appropriate work rate that suits and enhances your current standard of running fitness, and it may take time to do a 'number' of reps. While many people are similar, no two people are exactly the same. Improvement doesn't happen overnight, be patient, initially try not to hurt yourself too much – pain is a huge de-motivator, if it hurts too much you might not come back, what a waste!

My current philosophy regarding Park Runs is that they are a wonderful fun event, somewhere you can go, smile, enjoy, and in time begin to look forward to future communal get-togethers which have much to offer in terms of health and improved fitness, they're free, and you need a pair of shoes, 'you' cover 5km in whatever fashion you like, and you are one in a huge, but nevertheless minority in the world who can cover 5k in an energetic fashion – terrific! Well done.

Finally, a few chosen words from an old war horse of an athlete.

- Keep a training/exercise diary, and log down all your exercise sessions, a personal diary can be a real motivator, as well as allowing you to see at a glance how far you've come, perhaps since that first tentative step. If you need help (advice), your diary is like a personal CV, showing exactly where you were and indeed where you are now; as such they can help you go forward. As I've said before *'if I don't know where you've been, it becomes mighty difficult to take you somewhere else'*!

- Contrary to popular belief, the first lap is often harder than the last. It's the uncomfortable 'transition' phase from walking to jogging which is the culprit, as well as some 'mind games' resulting in a bit of negative 'self-talk'. From the off, you get into a bit of *oxygen debt* – that's because you've accelerated from standing start to a run and it takes the body just a little while to accustom itself to the increased effort. A decent 'warm-up' can assist here. A very short while later your body will have made the change/transition, and with it you've become more comfortable – bear with it. What I've learned over many years is that almost everyone 'raises their game' in terms of energy expenditure in the last 100 metres of a run or the last mile of a cycling competition – we all find just a little more energy... now where does it come from?

- My nana used to say to me when I was small after we'd got on a bus *'sit at the back, son, you get a longer ride for the same fare!'* What I'm getting at is this, on some enthusiastic days when you attend the Park Run and you're feeling good, stand a little closer to the front. The effect is the same as the bus journey but in reverse – you aren't running as far as you would if you were at your customary position near the rear. A Personal Best time by just one solitary second is still a Personal Best!

- If you aren't fit on a Monday, it's unlikely you'll be fit on the Saturday either. Take it easy the last two or three days before a 'concerted effort' if you are going for a personal best time, don't get there tired from too much the previous days is all I mean. I've been there countless times, took me a long time to work it out, training too hard right up to the event is a needless waste of energy. I was so often just too enthusiastic and it was self-defeating!

- Eat little amounts before your timed run, you have several days of fuel tucked comfortably inside your tum, and this 5km is not going to burn it all up. For years a marathon runner's breakfast consisted of Bread and Jam, easy to digest and tried and tested. Eating like there is a famine on the horizon will do you no favours. In contrast to food, force yourself to hydrate (the shade of your urine is a sound indicator, clear colour is best); water is best although a cup of tea or coffee will do you no harm, even on cool/cold days you will perspire – unless you're a celeb of course, they perspire neat Chanel No 5, and Old Spice aftershave, because they are all so beautiful, even the men! You mean handsome, don't you? No, I mean yummy, beautiful!

- Last one. I do believe this by the way. Smile and look jolly, it's referred to occasionally as *facial feedback hypothesis,* your facial expression does affect your body, neck down, be positive!

To my 'reluctant' models, Clare, Gill, Lindsay, Lisa, Judith and Sean. You are the epitome of the casual, keep fit people, combining busy lives whilst in the process managing to keep fit and always with a smile – a great example to us all. I'd buy you a lemonade but alas I can't catch you!

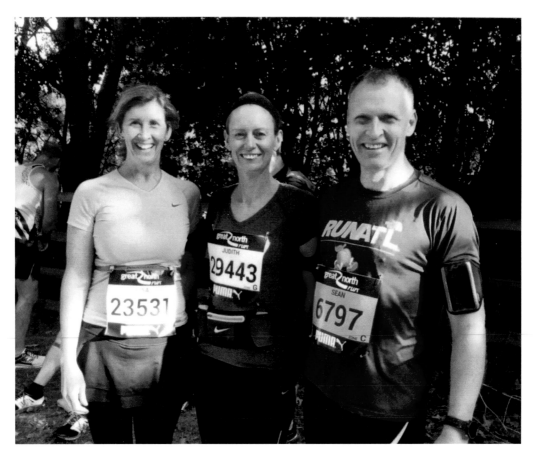

Lisa, Judith and Sean. Still smiling after the run, can't be bad.

WEIGHT and STRENGTH TRAINING

The title of this book uses the word 'experiment'; as such here is some more personal physical training that fits somewhere within the terms of reference.

Looking back over all my many decades involved in sporting competition, I have almost always performed some form of resistance or strength training. We did a lot of strength work when I was in the Marines because arguably the activities we did in the commando role relied on 'sound' upper-body composition. When being transported on commando carriers to venues around the globe with a lack of any elaborate equipment on-board, and to maintain some level of fitness and body strength, we'd use our body as the resistance, so, press-ups, abdominal work in all its varying forms, dips, pull-ups, rope climbing, vaulting, stepping and so on were almost daily routines. My view is straightforward and that is: if you think strength work is good for you (and I believe it is) there is 'no excuse' for not doing it. Those few exercises outlined above require little in the way of ingenuity and can be performed anywhere and additionally they take up very little of your time, they can even be done in the ten minutes it takes you to run your monthly bath! I was once on board a ship called HMS Fearless (it had a 'flat bottom', 'a bit like mine', terrible going through the notorious Bay of Biscay, oh god!) with Y Company 45 commando, while travelling out to take part in NATO exercises in the Mediterranean. The conditions were cramped, but below deck there was a helicopter; leading down to it there was a ramp of about 20 metres in length, and I can recall running up and down this slippery steep ramp while doing strength work in between the sprints (a form of circuit training), with an American Marine Officer as it happens, while being 'egged on' by a group of sadistic 'spectators', which as you can imagine led to a very 'competitive' workout – I won – he stopped before me! Thinking back, that was probably the trip where we also sailed into Gibraltar and I won a race to the top of the 'rock' and back down! Would I have won it if I hadn't kept fit during the journey? I don't know, but it didn't do me any harm. I can also vaguely recall being in some foreign land and standing in a sodden wet trench in the dark trying to keep my 7.62 SLR dry while at the same time doing press-ups and jogging on the spot, probably as much to do with keeping warm as trying to maintain some strength. Then later on, when I'd left the mob, I worked in three different Sports Centres and I would have real issues walking past the weights rooms without going in and doing three sets of bench pressing etc. A while later I got really lucky and my job with the police for 24 years meant I had a gym within 10 metres of my office – how could I refuse. **However, what I never did was sacrifice a swim, cycle or run session for a strength training workout.** As mentioned, I've done them all my life. As I write, I've very recently injured my Achilles 'again', as such I've been on the bike instead of my preferred (at the moment) running and as usual I can't feel this painful injury whist pedalling even during a normal two-hour ride, and, call it 'habit', I've finished off with press-up, dips, abdominal work, bicep curls and shoulder press. All facilitated using basic dumbbells in our utility followed by some mandatory stretching. Now, did my competitive sports reap the benefits of the added strength gained during these supplementary exercises? You know what, with a huge degree of honesty – I really don't know! Would I have won all those competitions if I hadn't done the additional strength work? My gut response is 'probably', but? Regardless, I suppose the exercises I've done for years were nothing if not complementary, or in certain respects necessary in view of all my occupational roles, some of which were supervising thousands of exercises as a Physical Training Instructor or practising Martial Artist.

Here is some 'condensed' information some might find useful.

There's no doubt that weight training is an important activity for measuring or improving strength, but it is only part of physical training. In isolation (for the 'athlete') it has limited value. No one ever died of a weak bicep muscle! But the heart? Now that's a different story.

What follows is basic, nevertheless! Weight training can be used to good effect for various purposes; these may include:

'Specific' weight training

Can be used as an aid in improving aspects of your individual sport or pastime (yes, even gardening) e.g. cycling, swimming, rugby, rowing, football, and most other miscellaneous athletic events.

Rehabilitation

Weight training can be used as an aid in strengthening specific areas such as knees, or calves following an Achilles injury, other areas having been developed through aerobic, anaerobic and flexibility programmes.

As part of a basic Exercise routine and general tone-up

Weight training is useful when aimed at complementing all-round fitness.

As mentioned previously, all training should be consistent, progressive, and specific (to the aim). So starting at a level which is 'comfortable' is really essential. That's not necessarily easy, because many of us have a competitive nature, and some gym users compete with each other and some don't know there're doing it, sometimes it's a 'macho' thing, and weights can be destructive in that regard. Trying to match the efforts of your 'neighbour 'in terms of the weight used or the amount of reps is folly! Be your own person and in others you'll encourage intrigue, and respect, rather than apathy, which sits alongside uniformity. I have an instinctive respect for those who buck the trend and manage their own training session with a degree of intelligence as well as energy; *less (as the saying goes) is often more!*

As with most forms of physical training, don't be tempted to 'rush' things, I've been there too many times myself – you'll look the same tomorrow as you do today, but in two months' time?!!! Remember all physiological improvement comes about during the rest and recovery phase following the exercise – no rest – no improvement. Fatigue, as happens all too often, may be responsible for the pending injury.

Weight training can place considerable stress on certain parts of the body and this stress can be magnified by poor technique, so again, show your intelligence and ASK FOR HELP, from an employee whose job it is to help, not from the person next to you which may turn out to be the worst decision of your new athletic life. It isn't the weight training apparatus which causes the injury, it's the manner in which the individual uses it – be careful!

It's obvious but I'll say it anyhow, this book is not all about weight training, but I am comfortable including some within it as there are clearly benefits from the inclusion if they are done for the right reason. For athletes who compete at events of 5km upwards, the benefits are not as important as the 'power' athletes, i.e. sprinters and field event exponents. My advice is that endurance athletes should concentrate more on doing *'strength endurance' exercises, that is the use of lighter weights with more repetitions, and sprinters, and field events as well as cycling should clearly be using larger weights with fewer reps and that's because 'power' is needed for the more explosive-type events.*

I personally don't like people below the age of 'at least' 16 'tampering' with weights – growing and developing bodies are very vulnerable in relation to injury, especially whilst they are developing. If I had a son or daughter considering the use of weight training, perhaps as a supplementary exercise, I would say categorically *'not yet, how about using 'body-weight instead, that's press-ups, dips, step-ups etc'.* Regardless, subject knowledge and expert on the shop floor assistance should be at hand. For the novice, here are some familiar used terms which you need to be conversant with:

How much should I lift? First thing to do is get a sensible, mature and physically able 'spotter' to act as your safety device. A spotter is a person who will act immediately as your support in the case of you getting into difficulty. *It is dangerous to do certain exercises without a spotter.* Remember we are all so very different and this is such a huge issue regarding weight training. The method I used when I had a novice to work with was like this: Using 'bench press' (a great all-rounder) with me spotting, we'd begin with a light weight and complete one full up and down repetition; if that was easy, then cautiously I'd add on a little more weight and repeat, continue with this system until the operator could lift the end weight just once; we'd then call that their maximum weight. Following this exercise, we would decide whether the aim was to improve 'strength endurance' or to increase their 'absolute strength' (power). If the aim was to improve strength endurance, we'd select a weight at a percentage of the maximum push, e.g. if their max push was 100kilo (I'm keeping it simple for this example) we could work at 50% of the max so in this case 50kilos and we'd then do between 15-25 reps. If the aim was more to do with 'absolute strength' we'd cautiously work at 75-95 kilos but with fewer reps, i.e. 3-10 depending on the chosen weight. Now it's important to say at this stage that the amount of reps can rise and of course they can fall; in so doing the weights are tailor made for each individual. See definition of reps and sets below.

A rep (repetition) is 'one' full movement (push, pull, lift) from start to finish. It works the same way for press-ups, i.e. one press-up equals one rep.

A set is 'several' reps put together as in a bundle i.e. 25 x 10kilos (that's strength endurance) OR 3-5 reps of much heavier weight (that's absolute strength).

So for the purpose of recording your specific workout in your training diary you could record it as – 25 x 25kilos bench press, or 3 sets of 25k bench press, meaning you've done 75reps in total, split into 3 sets and an appropriate rest/recovery between sets. Or, 3 sets of 10 x 80kilos three-quarter squats.

The more detail I write, the more uncomfortable I become, that's because writing so much detail has to be interpreted correctly – so again please use this brief info as a guide only. My intention is not to create endless advice on weight orientated exercise, rather to expand on what is on the menu within the scope of 'exercise', so bear that in mind. *Remember, as stated in an early chapter, this book is primarily 'for the ordinary by the ordinary', not specifically for the accomplished or specialist athlete!*

What are the best exercises? Well, there isn't 'one', and that's because there are loads of 'options' and they all have differing assets depending on your aim. However, bench press is a very good upper body all-rounder, because it utilises the chest, the shoulders front and rear, the back of the upper arms and the forearms. It doesn't use the front of the arms too much, so a bicep curl exercise could follow. Some work 'antagonistically', which means you work on opposite or opposing muscle groups – bicep curl followed by triceps extension, see? Back and front, so you create an equal balance. I've deliberately avoided using more technical terms such as pectorals, latissimus dorsi, or gluteus maximus. If you want more specialist advice I'm sure there are countless books out there, but a good 'sensible' trainer is worth their weight in 'steel'!

Finally, my advice is simple, and keeping within the terms of reference of this book, strength training is valuable, but depending on your aims, try not to get 'obsessed' with weight training unless it's for weight lifting competitions. With athletes wishing to complement their endurance or power for sprinting then there are benefits; however, remember what I said previously – I never aborted a swim, cycle or running session for a weight training session, but I've 'always' found time and space for press-ups, abdominal work, dips, etc. Even today – 28/2/2021, I rode for two hours very hard (lovely windless morning), then on conclusion I spent approximately 25 minutes doing Bar press-ups, dips, curls and military press, loads of differing abdominal and core work together with stretching (head to toe), so what did I end up with? Legs and cardio worked on the bike, as well as upper body maintenance through the resistance exercises, abdominals and core, and stretching to finish, now that's a pretty comprehensive all round physical work-out! **Complemented 'of course' by sound nutrition.**

<u>**REMEMBER THIS PLEASE.**</u> **IF THIS BOOK IS AT ALL 'DIFFERENT' THEN IT'S WORTH ME SAYING AGAIN,** 'I've done this sort of thing all my life, I'm still doing it, and I'm 70 years old'. The title I'm considering using includes the word 'experiment' – so far at least the experiment has gone on for 70 years, and touch wood I'm still in good nick – apart from a recent Achilles strain picked up on Tuesday running, and you know why I've damaged it? Because I run too bloody quick and too bloody well long! But I love running, so now I'll recover wisely, and then carry on. But the switched on athlete should be continually learning, and adjusting their exercise programme based to a degree on their past personal history!

Having talked about Aerobic and Anaerobic exercise as well as Strength work, put them together in one training session and you have another form of exercise:

CIRCUIT TRAINING

Circuit training is acknowledged as being one of the most effective methods of developing 'all-round' fitness. When performed correctly, it incorporates all the major elements of fitness (with differing degrees of emphasis).

AEROBIC (cardio-vascular conditioning primarily stamina endurance), ANAEROBIC (speed and power), STRENGTH (primarily in the case of circuits – strength endurance, i.e. the ability to repeat an activity many times), and FLEXIBILITY (to develop or maintain a range of movement).

ALSO, YOU CAN DO A FORM OF CIRCUITS 'ANYWHERE' FROM A SITTING ROOM, BACK GARDEN OR YARD, FOOTBALL FIELD, BEACH, PARK OR THE LUXURY OF A GYMNASIUM.

Equipment can be anything robust enough to stand up to the rigours of the exercises and the weight of the participants. Dumbbells are great, a bar bell allows many permutations, medicine balls, benches. chairs (for step-ups and a variety of press-ups) are all useful.

A typical example of a potential circuit:

We'll keep it simple. We have decided on five exercises in our circuit; press-ups*, sit-ups, step-ups, tricep dips, and squat-thrusts (two arms/upper body, two legs (and cardio) and abdominals.

Warm-up to slowly prepare the body for the forthcoming exertions.

Station 1 = 10 press-ups, walk or jog to station 2 = step-ups, that's 5 on each leg, walk or jog to station 3 = 10x sit-ups, walk or jog to station 4, and 10 x bench dips, and finally to complete the circuit finish off with 10 x squat thrusts. Walk around for 5 minutes to recover then commence on your second circuit with the option of maybe losing two reps on each activity.

Cool down gradually and have a natter!

The permutations are endless, for example you can use your timepiece (stopwatch) to control the amounts, i.e. 20 seconds on each exercise, before moving on; this way you avoid any 'bunching up' of people because you all move on together.

Despite the name 'circuits' they don't have to be performed using a circle, you can go in straight lines, which means it's easier to add on more walking or running between exercises.

A potential negative with circuits, if using equipment, is that one size doesn't fit all, e.g. a 10k dumbbell is great for some but too light or too heavy for others, whereas the use of your body as the resistance is simpler and safer, so press-ups, bench dips, squat thrusts, step-ups etc are a much easier prospect in terms of management.

To Carl and Mel, 'that's the way to do it' – and always with a smile on your face, good to know you, well done!

CROSS TRAINING

During the 70s, and early 80s running with Morpeth Harriers I regularly trained in excess of 100 miles a week in preparation for athletic competition. The 'positive' side of such dedicated, consistent, and specific training was 'good' performances and Championship medals. The 'negative' downside was fairly consistent injury problems caused by the 'overuse syndrome' or the commonly used phrase Repetitive Use Syndrome (RUS).

In 1983, following a magazine article, I changed direction and moved into the swim, bike, run sport of Triathlon. My enthusiasm was such that I very quickly proceeded to train three times daily, six or seven days a week. A normal day would be: 7.00am 3000 metre swim, 8-10 mile run at lunchtime, and a 30-40 mile cycle in the evening, that's 25 hours each week, combined with a 37-hour working week.

The positive side of all this, was a member of the Great Britain Triathlon team for ten years (and plenty of trips abroad), several times British Champion, holder of records and European medals! However, the biggest bonus was NO INJURIES!!! For 12 years of involvement in triathlon I was never laid up with injury and that's despite the severity of my training regime.

This chapter is on 'CROSS TRAINING'. Balance is crucial in exercise. Invariably weight trainers train with weights, runners run, swimmers swim, and footballers play five-a-side. The by-product is an imbalance of strengths and weaknesses, i.e. weight trainers with no aerobic capacity and runners with no strength.

Are they really fit? I would argue 'ONLY IN PARTS'!! Be careful you don't shine the exterior (chassis) too much; beauty is skin deep. The interior (engine and fuel lines) is more important, muscular types may look attractive? However, it's the cardio that keeps you alive.

So, what is Cross Training and how can I use it?

Cross Training can be defined as a group of activities which when used together, help produce an individual who possesses an 'all-round balance' of physical fitness.

Within the confines of physical prowess certain qualities are desirable, in general terms; these are strength, stamina, speed and flexibility. Differing degrees of all four areas are desirable depending on the individual sport or aim.

Whatever sports or activities we partake in, we could all concede that from the specific sport we will gain certain qualities. Few individual activities will include the four areas outlined above so, invariably, we end up with an imbalance – typically, a marathon runner who can't do press-ups or vice versa a weight lifter or body builder who can't run. Cross training is a modern-day term which simply implies that we take part in several training activities with the intention of creating 'total fitness'. The aim of total fitness is to minimise our specific weaknesses whilst maximising our strengths.

The benefits of cross training principles are:

- Increased endurance (see chapter on aerobics)
- Increased speed of movement (see chapter on anaerobic activity)
- Increased strength (see chapter on weight training)
- And increased mobility and flexibility (see chapter on mobility/flexibility)

Which exercises are best?

For all four elements combined in one, three activities spring to mind for an all-round training effect: rowing, circuit training and possibly swimming (although there is little in the way of bone strengthening in the non-weight bearing activity of swimming). But for the keep fit enthusiast there is little doubt that combinations of exercises are best.

A very simplified week's training could look similar to the following, although clearly there are numerous permutations:

Monday = swim, Tuesday = weight training, Wednesday = jogging/stretching, Thursday = circuit training, Friday = Badminton/Squash, Saturday = Rowing/Stepping/cycling/stretching, Sunday = Recreational walk.

The vigilant amongst us will no doubt say: 'Hey, no rest days, that's asking for trouble!' Well, one of the real pluses of cross-training is the variety, and primarily because we are constantly changing the emphasis of physical stress from one body area to another, we are quite naturally also inadvertently allowing physiological recovery. An example of cross training leading to competition is as follows:

ULTRA FIT COMPETITIONS

Now they required 'cross training' to simulate the content of the competitions.

At some point around the year 2000, I read an article in a magazine about ultra-fit competitions. At the time I had finished with triathlon and was simply working-out every day with no real aim apart from keeping fit; as such I was often supervising circuit training sessions and using the gym apparatus at work. I was missing the adrenalin that naturally comes with sporting competitions and so, having read the article, I decided to set my sights on the event at

Wolverhampton – if nothing else it would be something new and the event would no doubt act as a motivator to work hard at something different for a while. My training was all 'cross-training', running, rowing, stationary cycling sessions, stepping and a wide variety of core and strength work; we even had ropes in the HQ gym which I had barely used since my days in the Marines. I became very 'able' with an impressive (especially for a 50 year old) all-round level of fitness, which as I remember made me feel particularly good. As always a lot of thought went into my preparation and my training was tailor made for the intended event, although some of the competition apparatus varied somewhat from what I had available at HQ and a gym I used at weekends at Red Row.

And so, at 6am, on the 19th May 2001 I made the lengthy journey down to RAF Cosford near to Wolverhampton to compete in the National 'X' Zone Grand Finals. The event took place in a massive RAF aircraft hangar and consisted of 10 'consecutive' aerobic, anaerobic, and strength exercises. There were several 'waves' of competitors, 10 or 12 of us in a line with each of us delegated an RAF PTI to count our repetitions and to ensure techniques were by the book. The event began with a 2km recumbent cycle followed immediately by the following further nine exercises: 50 x press-ups, 2.5km treadmill run (on a 3% incline), 1,200kg (60 x 20kgs) seated shoulder press, 1,500metre row (concept 2), 50 x sit-ups, 2 x 12' rope climbs, 45 x floors on a stepper, 4km cycle (no.8 setting), and culminating with Medicine ball shuttle run. I won my age group; I was 50 at the time. I remember the event as an 'extremely' hard work-out which pushed me, as I remember, to the limit! Training for the event was a daily commitment and the end result as you can imagine was a finely toned all-round athlete. I've detailed the above info just as a guide and to give a practical insight into the rigours of 'Cross-Training'!

So in summary, what we can develop is an interesting and varied all-round schedule resulting in TOTAL FITNESS. *Remember all the above are 'very simple' examples, you can of course alter everything and mould the schedule to best suit you the individual; above all, remain motivated and keep active while remaining injury-free!.*

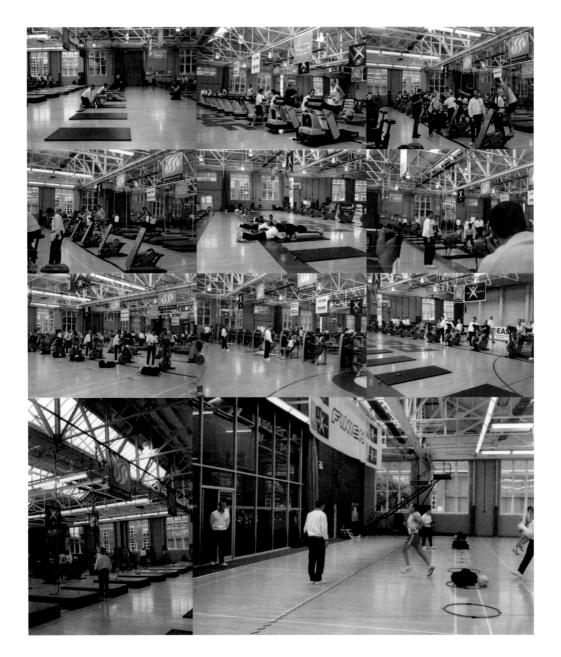

Super fit at 50 (I'm in red shorts)

To Gary Hall, my gratitude, Gary, a calm, interested professional, reliable friend and fellow athlete, wishing you a long career as athlete and professional! Thanks for all your valued help.

Injury and Illness

Writing reams on these two topics would include a lot of replication, stuff that's been done a million times before, and that was one area (obvious replication) I was hoping to avoid as far as reasonably possible in putting this book together, so as such I'll keep this subject 'very' brief.

I have been very lucky with *general health*, and as a child *'luck'* really does come into the equation of personal health, because we're all dealt a hand that has little to do with us in the womb, if it's a bad hand – well it couldn't be seen as our fault. When we're born the hand we hold has little to do with 'what we deserve' and more to do occasionally with parentage combined with a mixture of either good fortune or bad luck. In any order you like, wealth, intelligence, god-given talent, support and 'health' are part of the package we inherit or avoid, and in my formative years with the latter although it was normal for lads, I took some boyhood knocks; however, the main thing was I was given the supreme gift of good health and was never ill. After those early years, however, we gradually begin to take responsibility for the life you lead and all the repercussions and bonuses that gradually develop with it, and so I think later on we *'make your own luck'* as far as health is concerned; as such we either retain it or we randomly give it away. I learned very quickly as an athlete that 'general health' complemented athletically orientated physical prowess, however, and regardless, like most young men I occasionally revelled in a good social life and so I got drunk, chased women, acted the goat and enjoyed youth for what it is, a potentially wonderful free from restraint period where it seems all things are possible and every time you fall, well, you pick yourself up, dust yourself off and quickly move on with a smile to the next spill!

With the usual fairly common **illnesses** we all get from time to time, and I'm talking every day colds and the resulting cough I always seem to get with them; well I simply ignored them as the inconvenience they were and still are and continue to exercise/train throughout their duration and being outside in the fresh Northumbrian countryside is a great pick-me-up tonic, although I may reduce the exercise intensity. I have 'never' taken chemist type medication or pills (for 35/40 years I've never touched codeine, aspirin, paracetamol, ibuprofen or whatever, and only once taken as prescribed by the Doc antibiotics for an insect bite and resulting infection, I don't need them – nor have I ever sipped 'relief' type products in my life, although I can recall my mother giving me, when I was very young, half an aspirin in a teaspoon with a bit of jam on top! Now with regard to the latter and whichever way you look at it 40 years is a long 'experiment' and I'm still here, still healthy and superbly fit! I have written about pills and medication before, and my opinion is that they are just too convenient and accessible, and most people are by nature both habitual as well as followers – as such we are easily influenced and we always believe that someone somewhere always knows better, well, doctors get colds as well, I wonder if they are as quick to feed themselves a variety of countless pills and medicines they so willingly feed others?

What I have learned about **injuries*** is that as soon as you put someone into physical motion there is a risk and injuries for the athlete are 'almost inevitable', I mean show me an athlete who has never had an injury and I'll show you a celeb who has an aversion to publicity, they come with the terrain and the harder you physically work, the more you tread a vulnerable path, and once you stumble and are laid up, well, there are absolutely no quick fixes. I have had all sorts of injuries, all *soft tissue* and the vast majority were due to *'overuse'*, and with me, the activity of 'running' was the devil! Achilles, glutes, shin-splints, knees, calves, quads, groin, feet, and ankles, were all running-related! I have never had broken bones apart from my nose, I also had occasional facial bruising when I boxed, which I'd put up with because they both (bruising and a crooked nose) seemed to make people laugh, and if I could give some poor sod a bit of joy in their otherwise sad life well so be it!!

How do you prevent injuries?

Whilst it is 'easy' to continually succumb to a wide array of injuries (and for many of them I know where they come from – they are seldom mysterious), I believe it is potentially much easier to avoid them than accumulate them, but as with most things there is an art to remaining injury free, and that art as I've referred to it derives around 'discipline'. Athletes are their own worst enemies, ambition and regular bouts of success are the nemesis (the goddess of retribution!) – the better we get the harder we try. The more successful we become, the more we pile on the workload, we are the never ending optimists and *more is better is the mantra we follow,* and the more we do in terms of physical work the more likely it becomes that an injury will be lurking ready to stop you dead in your athletic tracks; additionally the more you do in terms of speed and excessive distance, the greater the injury severity will be and the longer the self-imposed resting and recovery quarantine will take.

The athlete is a fit gambler; and the only difference between the two (athlete and gambler) is that athletes use a track and the gambler uses a casino, but both parties can be on a par in terms of blind ambition, and both these are always ready to travel the extra yard in search of the ultimate win! Additionally, both gamblers are a hair's breadth away from throwing all their gains away and leaving with nothing. Gamblers are often addicts – as are athletes – common sense and discipline are regularly absent within our make-up! The more driven we are the more foolish we can become! As a coach, just try reeling in your athlete when he/she is in good form and winning, yet there is a very thin dividing line between being super fit and being injured and backing off for a very short while could be the cleverest thing you've ever done.

What's the answer?

You'd quickly ridicule me if I gave '5 do's and 5 don'ts' whilst concluding with 'follow my advice and you'll never be injured again'! Now that is cow's crap – and enough of it to mulch many acres of prime agricultural land!!! Remember

I said somewhere that within sport there are no answers – only possibles, and that of course is the intrigue that keeps us continually searching and believing!

KEEP IT SIMPLE; I'll get certified for this!

YOU DON'T GET INJURED WHEN YOU'RE RESTING! YOU RARELY GET INJURED WHEN YOU ARE TRAINING EASY, I'VE ALSO DISCOVERED THAT YOU GET INJURED FAR LESS WHEN YOU ADD ON ANOTHER PHYSICAL DISCIPLINE *DESIGNED TO 'COMPLEMENT'* YOUR CARDIO SYSTEM WHILST ALLEVIATING THE OBVIOUS MUSCULAR STRESS AND PRESSURE APPLIED TO YOUR LEGS (AND ELSEWHERE DEPENDING ON YOUR ACTIVITY). TRIATHLON INVARIABLY SUITED ME, I WAS RARELY LAID UP WITH INJURY WITHIN THAT SPORT ALTHOUGH GOD KNOWS I TRAINED AND COMPETED LIKE A PERSON POSSESSED!! Few ever trained as I did and to a degree still do, in fact if there were Olympic medals for effort, I'd have a houseful!

All my injuries derived from running – either **running too much, too fast, and too often!** I 'never' got injured on the bike and I've done umpteen – thousands and thousands of miles – I never got injured swimming even when it was regularly seven days each week, although that water-based sport sent me very close to a place where I'd silently and regularly question my sanity such was the relentless boring slog of going endlessly up and down a tiled prison like chasm at 6.30am – before work!

I have also wondered a million times whether you always recover 100% from an injury, even when you believe it is long gone. My own left Achilles is the reminder if needed that that particular gremlin was never that far away. Injuries, as defeatist as it sounds, are simply repaired by time; although I have rarely tried them, creams and ointments are in my opinion are surplus to requirements, you'll heal just as quick without them and save a bob or two. If you disagree, think about the possibility of the Placebo effect, a real positive belief in all things tried is essential. ICE, I am quite confident, has real positive issues and it's free.

So, if you want progress in your sport or recreational activity whilst also creating longevity, accept with a great deal of discipline that the best panacea is simple REST (active and total), both are so incredibly crucial and should be placed in your training programme with the same diligence and degree of importance as the physically demanding elements!! REST is not a weakness.

*Back to triathlon after a 20 year break! Where there's a will there's a way!

In 2014 at 63 years of age, I decided to return to triathlon – why? INTRIGUE! Racing on the bike saw me mingling with triathletes at local cycle races, the triathletes often entered Time Trial events as a means of improving their tri' biking; now comparing my cycling with theirs (many were less than half my age) I was for the most part much quicker. Out of nowhere, on the 6th January 2014 I went swimming and swam 100 lengths front crawl, my first decent swim for 20 years commenting in my diary *'no bother – could have gone on'* and so began my 're-entry' into triathlon training and competition. With triathlon, of course, you have to run as well as swim and cycle, so on the 20th Jan I ran for 20 minutes at the beach with a 10 minute walk at the end for a cool down, my first run for years, although I would hastily add I was still super-fit. The end of the month my diary totals are logged as 10 swim sessions, 21 bike sessions and 10 jogs (legs stiff and sore from running). From the end of January to the end of February there were no further runs, comments – bad back, tender calves, hamstrings stiff, Achilles very tender and stiff, and glutes 'sore'! All the way through the 2014 training diary there are huge gaps where running was absent. I'll not bore you with the specific details, and regardless on the 8th June I took part in my first triathlon since 1994 and finished 20th from 250 entries and had the 3rd fastest bike split! RUNNING in my diary says: *Pleased to get through it but legs felt fine!*

Why am I even mentioning all this? Simply because it sits well in this chapter where I am referring to 'injuries'. A relatively short time later after several 'months' of struggle and in 2015 only months after struggling 'so badly' and repeatedly contemplating whether to stop this *folly*, well, I ran 18m 57s for the 5km Park Run at Druridge Bay. *Never say die* (as always a

personal mantra with me). I had gone from novice 'elderly' always injured runner to 2nd placings and from 57 Park Runs to date I've averaged 19m 47s and that's from 63 to 69 years of age, before the Covid-19 mayhem for the cancellation of the Park Run events lasting for almost 18 months right up to today.

IS THERE A LEARNING CURVE EVEN AT 70? ABSOLUTELY! Once again, solely based on my *'personal logged experiences', stay with it*; but, explore the *alternatives and there are many, and* don't keep doing the same repetitive stuff that always results in injury – wise-up!!! When incorporating running into your training/exercise programme experiment with stretching (be careful), rehab work (you could do worse than book a session or two with Gary Hall), use 'cheap' first aid treatments such as RICE, change of footwear, self-massage, change running surfaces, don't run out five miles because if you begin to feel abnormal tenderness or pain – well, you have to run the five mile back, so stay local or do circuits round a two-mile loop and be extra careful with hills in particular running down on concrete! AND INCORPORATE WELL THOUGHT OUT REST DAYS AND EVEN EXTENDED REST PERIODS.

And for something totally different and nothing at all to do with this publication:

I was looking for an 'elusive' word before in my little dictionary and I found this, which has tickled my self-professed occasional weird sense of humour!

The word I uncannily came across was **Tit!** And the explanation given by the presumed intellect who is the proud possessor of a multitude of academic degrees including English was: a *female breast OR a despicable stupid person (I wonder who he was thinking of)!*

I can't stop smiling as I see the author sitting writing that interpretation down – if a Royal Marine had written that he'd be straight over the sea and back out to the Falklands 'till he got better'!

As you will have discovered, in this book, I've used space to record personal sentiment regarding people who have gained my total respect – here's another!

To Mike Bateman, a genuine colossus on the North Eastern Athletics scene, for what seems like centuries. My hat goes off to you, Mike, with so much respect – what would they have done without you? You've been terrific!

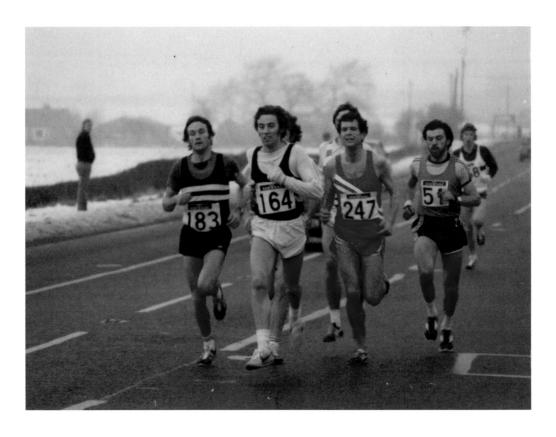

Mike Batemen and me Morpeth - Newcastle. I was in good company running with Mike Bateman (164), a great club runner for Morpeth.

WHAT ABOUT COACHES, AND COACHING ATHLETES?

As mentioned previously, I have never had a coach in my entire life – I didn't avoid coaches, but nobody asked me, as such, it just didn't happen. I joined Morpeth Harriers as a 15 year old in 1966; even then at that informative age I wasn't part of a coaching set-up. I read books, dreamt, watched others and copied. As detailed in my autobiographies, my dad left home when I was 8 or 9, and from that point onwards we didn't have a car, and I live at Widdrington, which is in the middle of nowhere and seven miles east of Morpeth. So I attended Morpeth Harriers by bus, 'if' my mother had the fare; if she didn't I biked through. I rarely thought about it, although returning was a struggle, especially pedalling a squeaky little gear-free bike up the notorious Whorral Bank. As far as racing went, I was occasionally picked up at Widdrington's Co-op by either Tommy Horne or Peter Carmichael (I am still indebted to you both and always will be – truly wonderful people). The Harriers met then as indeed they do now on Monday evenings; additionally in my youth in those days, they met early on a Sunday morning for the week's traditional long endurance run. Now in those days buses didn't run from Widdrington before 11am on a Sunday, so I wheeled my bike out of the 'coal house' around 6.30am, dusted the coal dust off the seat and biked the seven miles through, then ran up to 12 miles or so with the seniors, before pedalling the seven miles home. After a hastily gobbled down Sunday lunch I then played football for most of the afternoon on the bottom green; we'd often keep going till it got too dark to continue. I joined the Royal Navy/Royal Marines at 15 years of age, got on a train 'single crewed' at Widdrington – job done, almost! And although I represented the Corps in four sports, I still had no coaching, apart from 'supervision' and a few tips in Boxing. In my mid-twenties, after leaving the Marines, I returned to Morpeth Harriers and resumed my self-coached lifestyle whilst winning amongst other things the North Eastern Counties Marathon title. The North East at that time (Gateshead was a hugely successful club, McLeod was at Elswick and Mr Cram was at Jarrow) almost 'ruled the world' (I'm not kidding) as far as distance running went (and so it was a good title to win). In my early 30s I moved into the world of Triathlon and won many British Championship titles and additional European medals with good placings in the World Champs. Twelve years later I finalised my triathlon years with an 8th place in the British Championships in Guernsey (I was 43 then) and proceeded to race bikes for the next 12 years or so and won at least 75 races. Throughout it all – well, I was never coached or assisted in any way apart from some sponsorship from Puma, Freewheel, and Terrapin wetsuits, as well as some GB kit!

What about coaching then? There are some sports where the early coaching needed to acquire sporting skills is of paramount importance. Learning 'motor skills' at a very early age are worth their weight in gold. Nobody forgets how to ride a bike or how to swim once the preliminaries are engrained! Sports such as athletic field events including the throws, the jumps and even the sprints need guidance and expertise to educate the finer technical parts of the activity, resulting in a finely schooled athlete complemented by energy saving skills. Swimming is another – learn the feel for the water at a young age and just like riding a bike it will be stored and become part of your long term memory. Martial Art activities are another that requires skill, that's hand and eye coordination combined with specific movement. The latter hand/eye co-ordination is also a huge part of 'ball' games. But running middle and long distances require (after the formative years) little in the way of technical skills. As mentioned, the young need guidance but after the mid-twenties, if you've received guidance for the last 10-plus years and you are reasonably intelligent, I think (and as I keep saying – it's only me) coaching is unnecessary, or perhaps useful only as having someone's experience to occasionally turn to when things aren't going according to plan and you respectfully ask a coach 'can I run something past you?'.

Middle and long distance running are the freest and most uninhibited of all activities; go back to our beginning, and out of the cradle, we instinctively begin our physically active life by crawling – **and them days we are always motivated**, when strong enough we get around to walking, and then we can't wait to run, and it's all in that order, no tuition required and more to the point it's natural and instinctive! The physiology of running is interesting and is similar to all activities, we've covered it earlier. Just like a car which has an engine and wheels, the body has similar components. The heart is the pump which supplies the body with the fuel, the fuel is transported in the blood stream via an abundance of blood vessels, and the legs and the arms are the wheels that produce the movement. The bigger and stronger the heart (the engine) the more fuel it can additionally transport, the stronger the legs and arms become, and the more efficient is the running machine, it all works together, the whole is better than the sum of parts, so even with running a 'holistic' approach is best.

In my professional life, I have supervised literally thousands of physical training sessions and countless self-defence training sessions, I did it for 24 years, almost every week; before that I was a multi-sports coach working in three separate sports centres. I also taught swimming for several years, BUT I have only been involved in coaching/training/advising (by request) with four athletes, despite being a club coach in every event from 800 metres right up to and including the marathon. In addition, I have several sports coaching qualifications including miscellaneous events such as trampoline, table tennis, and gymnastics, and I have a Black Belt in Tiaho-Jutsu. Three of the four athletes I coached/trained asked me for help and I couldn't refuse – the four are a delight, my son David, Ryan Green, Daniel Dixon and as I write Joe Dixon. I wasn't personally being selective, I didn't and never would ever dream of poaching athletes from other coaches, I was asked to help, and nodded my acceptance.

To clarify the above, all my life I have been a 'selfish' competitive athlete, an amateur in every sense of the word, a working family man, who has trained and competed consistently almost every year of my 70 year life, always in search of personal success, so how on earth could I have given the amount of time required to train other athletes and do them justice when my life was, and still is to a degree, so frenetically and utterly busy? Part of my success was due to being utterly selfish, there were never enough hours in the day to consider other athletes, but I have the greatest respect for others like Mike Bateman, Jim Alder, Tony Ward, Gordon Dixon, Archie Jenkins and 'others' who have almost given their lives to assist athletes reach their potential, you are truly wonderful!!

I have pointed out above that with some sports, coaching is essential, and 'all kids' need advice and supervision when they first enrol in sporting activities, because apart from the obvious skill acquisition there is also a health and safety responsibility issue which out-weighs everything. Whenever I discussed training with Ryan and Daniel, I made sure their parents were present, they needed to agree with my proposals, and had every right to voice any concerns they may have had due to my proposed methods.

Just a thought! Education within sports clubs: How terrific it would be for an athlete or 'former athlete' to be able to state in a later casual conversation, **'I learned that from my athletic club when I was 10!'**

I am on the periphery of clubs, I am a passive observer, not a criticiser, due to my non-involvement I have no right to criticise, and volunteer supervisory club staff are a truly wonderful group of people; however, there is more to it than the physical part, particularly amongst the young. Early education can last a lifetime, and there is a wonderful opportunity within sporting clubs of all persuasions to school and educate its members. In brief I am talking about diet/nutrition, personal hygiene (even bathing, teeth brushing, and cutting toe nails), what role suppleness can play or perhaps the inclusion of strength work and educating 'when appropriate' about fair play issues and sporting etiquette and basic life skills. And how about offering a 20 minute (once every couple of months) 'sitting down' session based on questions and answers?

Having said all of that, I have often been bemused as to why 'mature' distance running athletes feel a need to seek a coach. It is no secret that animosity has been rife in athlete/coaching circles. If an athlete fails to meet their anticipated standards, they will often leave their current coach and seek out another coach, yet the athlete will, on occasions, have been running for many years, and therefore it's fair to assume the runner is experienced, in all methods of training. The 'abandonment' of the often long-term coach seems like the athlete is to a degree blaming the coach for a lack of improvement. The activity which is running is fundamentally simple, what skill do you need to put one foot in front of another? How do you acquire stamina? How do you convert the stamina into added speed? What foods are best, pre, during, and after running? How do you remain injury-free? How do you extend your range of movement? How do you increase muscular strength without 'bulking' up? It's simple stuff. What I do believe is the more people an athlete surrounds themselves with, the more complex it all becomes, too many cooks. *On another more positive note, and despite what I've said, coaches can be an absolute godsend, as motivators, physicians, historians, and psychologists, they also see things the athlete doesn't, and they see it all objectively from a distance. For me I could tell when an athlete was running well because of their physical* running form, not effort, although for the athlete it was just another session, pretty much the same as the last; now if I could see when the athlete was running well, clearly with a bit of analysis I could also see when the session should be aborted because to continue would be at that time too risky.

I believe I was successful in sports as a self-coached athlete, because I knew myself inside out, thoroughly, and in-depth, I knew what I was good at and I knew my weaknesses, I went along the lines of if I failed it wasn't my coach's fault (I didn't have one), it wasn't because of fitness, motivation or lack of training, it was because I just wasn't good enough on the day, as such there were better athletes present, hats-off to them because sport doesn't carry anyone – if someone is winning they have worked for it and they don't find it easier than you, although it may look that way! The regrets I personally have are that I lost some events for various reasons, which I could have and should have won; as difficult as it is, it's all part of the game. I also to a degree lost some events which were mine to win, by a lack of the 'super' equipment others had – I'm talking bike!

What I dislike most about modern day 'competitive' sport is the occasional boredom factor that comes with knowing the outcome before the commencement. Knowing the result even before the whistle blows defies all logic. The financial differences between opponents ensures there's a huge gap between the 'haves' and the 'have-nots'! Some sports such as football, Formula one, rowing, tennis, equestrian, even Paralympics, are so far in front regarding support and riches that other teams and nations are simply in another league. Before the event even starts, we know what the outcome will be. In Formula 1, one of three will win despite the 40 other drivers taking part; in football four or five teams will reap all the competitive rewards as the rest are battling just to stay up as well as make the top five look good; tennis is the same – betting on anyone apart from the two or three favourites is folly, and don't we know who will lift the trophies at the end; it's sad, primarily because sport was at least partially designed to be above all fair and to be played on a level playing field, honesty, ethical issues, an unbiased degree of sporting fairness not influenced by wealth.

A little bit for the athlete – and still there are few answers!!

This book was not intended for the athlete as such, because there are countless books already out there, and all saying pretty much the same thing, and another one repeating the same would invariably make us, you and I, yawn. The only thing that may be interesting for the athlete in this publication is my 'longevity' because however you dress it up, that is 'unusual' (as is the way I did it), and there 'may' be things deriving from my lengthy career that others may find interesting, and primarily that's because I am not a 'gifted' athlete oozing talent, money or intelligence; I am just incredibly ordinary!

What I like about some athletic running events is that there are truly 'no answers' only possibles and probables, and isn't that just wonderful!! Wonderful because you never stop searching, even when successful (however you quantify that) you still search for improvement! What I mean is that 7x7 = 49 and 9+8 = 17, you spell Harris with two 'arse' and the previous are what you'd call 'answers' no debate they are irrefutably correct, however you argue the case the answers are simply fact and remain the same regardless of how you juggle them around. Now despite all the know-how in terms of athletic training principles and the many permutations that exist in forming a training plan, well – the final outcome is still mystical and will remain that way till the athlete 'calls time'! **What makes distance running interesting (especially for the athlete) is that *nothing is beyond a dream*. There have been numerous athletes (excuse this inappropriate term) who began running as a 'donkey' on the common, and through personal endeavour (discipline, consistency and self-belief) ended up an apparent 'thoroughbred' at Newmarket battling out 'neck and neck' a classic up the home straight. It's that unpredictability or uncertainty that keeps many of us athletes searching and trying. The other thing is, it's my belief that unlike so many other sports, even as an amateur runner with a job, you can still make it at the top level, you do that by getting up early before all others and running in the dark before work, you shower, have your porridge then go to work; at night on conclusion of your shift, you run again! What other sport, in today's world, allows you to progress without additional money, additional specialist equipment, arenas, velodromes, water or horses all complemented by two or three coaches to guide you.**

I said this wasn't for the athlete, so I'll not keep you hanging around, except to re-emphasise the point I make about a lack of answers. There have been a few 'very' successful coaches in the past who trained their athletes with vastly differing formulas. Percy Ceruty used local terrain to his advantage, particularly the sand dunes for strength work (running up) as well as leg speed work (running down) – he trained Herb Elliot to win the 1960 Rome Olympic 1500metres (he was never defeated in his career over either a mile or the 1500!). Then just over the ocean, there was Arthur Lydiard who had his middle-distance athletes doing extreme long distance endurance runs in the mountains. Both of these coaches were from the same part of the world, both extremely successful yet both had different methods of honing their athletes – which of them was right? They both were, once again there were no definitive answers - just maybes and possibilities. The biggest element in my opinion that 'may' lead to success for both coach and athlete is either knowing yourself (if self-coached) or knowing your athlete inside-out and being able to construct a training plan based on the uniqueness of the athlete and their realistic ambition.

Arguably my 'modest' success was all down to being 'self-coached', there was no one else to blame and no-one else to interfere, I had little in the way of money to juggle, a straightforward, cheap, functional diet, much of which was based on availability, an ability to put together many months of training and then to 'peak' at the right time, and an undeniable urge to see it all through without having the fear of 'wondering what could have been' had I not seen it all through!!

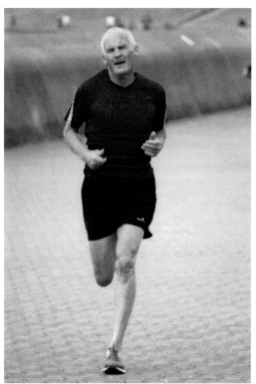 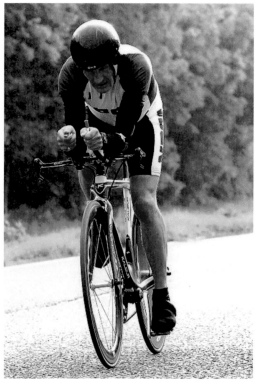

21 'consecutive' sub-20 minute park runs, even at 68...

...and a 10m, 23:18 time trial, at 70 years of age, on a course with 8 roundabouts.

OTHER TITLES BY MIKE HARRIS
TWO SELF PENNED AUTOBIOGRAPHIES

SIXTY YEARS AN ATHLETE

AND

SIXTY YEARS AN ATHLETE PART TWO
(just filling in the cracks)

All reviews were given '5 stars' except one from his Uncle in Australia which received a 4 star ha ha! Who needs friends eh? The reviews which follow are a small selection:

- *This book will have you not wanting to put it down. It's an incredible read that has been written brutally honestly by arguably the toughest triathlete to grace the planet ...bar no-one. Once you read this very honest account of what it takes to reach the top, you will simply sit back and wonder how it is even possible to train that hard while keeping down a full time job and family life too. Mikes hard work makes his racing speak for itself having been at the top of the tree for decades etc.*

- Bought for my husband who knows the author. He couldn't put it down, great down to earth book.

- *I started to read this book and could not put it down. What a guy. Talk about 'un-sung heroes', this is a man who never talks about himself in public. You have to read this book to get to know him. Well done Mike, can't wait to read your next book???*

- Very enjoyable read. What an incredible athlete.

- *Mike Harris is a North East sporting legend you probably never heard of. This book is a funny, entertaining and very enjoyable read, recounting Mike's life from early, modest beginnings to his rise and becoming the top British triathlete through sheer grit, effort and iron willed determination etc etc.*

- A must read book by a genuine sporting legend. Way back in the eighties when triathlon was a sport for 'nutters' Mike lead the way. With a grounding in endurance sport as a top class marathon runner, he turned to triathlon and applied his incredible worth ethic to being the best he could be which in his case was better than everyone else. Thirty years later he's still doing it, leaving seasoned competitors more than half his age trailing in his wake etc. etc.

- *Incredible insight into the mind and motivation of an elite amateur athlete. Funny, eclectic, nostalgic and engaging an entertaining and enjoyable book.*

- This book is a must have for anyone having an interest in sport. Mike pushes himself way beyond the limits in his pursuit of success, time and time again and does so in a quite matter of fact way. His training diaries are clearly unique and inspirational and left me in amazement etc.

- *Really enjoyable book, from growing up in a Northumberland mining village to life in the forces as well as being an athlete, and he's still going, saw him get a trophy at a triathlon last month.*

- Inspiring read. Fantastic insight into what amateur athletes can achieve while holding down full time jobs. A must read for all budding athletes be that triathletes to park runners, a brutally honest book.

- *This book is a great read. It is punchy, witty, irreverent and perfectly captures what it takes to compete at the highest level as a true amateur! A remarkable story written by a remarkable man.*

- On top of this is a good human story and an excellent read. If you want to view how to be an outstanding athlete and or be a triathlete this describes the effort, the determination, the understanding of yourself, this is the book for you. This has been done on a low budget and still received the reward it deserves.

- *This is not your normal athlete autobiography by any means! You could almost say that it's a window to the past when athletes in most sports were pure amateurs and fitted their training around full time jobs. Surely it is only in the last thirty years or so that the Corinthian attitude has given way to the professional ethos that would have been displayed on an olden day Rome arena etc.*

- Again, a fantastic read from a very engaging character. Motivational in everything he does without stopping to think too much about his own ego. I only have one problem with the books Mike Harris writes and that is I can't put them down, I look forward to part three!

- *A highly entertaining follow-on from the first book.*

- This is another great book written by an honest, straight-talking but humorous amateur athlete. I totally agree with another reviewer that you just can't put it down. It is written in such a way that if you are not an athlete, it explains how modern sport is so different to the past and Mike explains it very well and honestly. Brilliant reminiscing about life growing up and living in Northumberland makes this a great read and keeps you well entertained. Great job.

- *An irreverent memoir packed with humour! Mike Harris is much of an unsung hero with a palmares that Nationally funded athletes would envy – all on hard work and jam sandwiches. This second edition brings Mike's unique take on everything from politics to sport to domestic life. Keenly written it is like you are sitting across from him having a casual chat.*

- A second interesting, funny, inspirational book from amateur athlete Mike Harris, how he manages to cram so much living into twenty-four hours is beyond me! We constantly hear of top athletes failing drugs tests, well Mike will restore your faith in mankind! The man's a legend.

- *Not a keen reader by all accounts however as soon as I heard that Mike had written a book on his athletic career I knew I must buy it! It doesn't disappoint! From start to finish hearing what makes a top athlete tick and how he managed to train within normal working home is truly inspirational. Puts us all to shame, worth a read!*

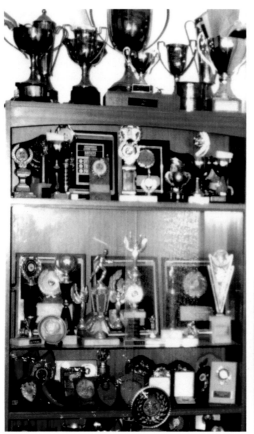

An amateur athlete, no money and no acclaim, but years of memories.

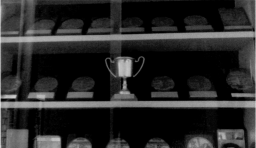

To Tom Maley, you opened doors for me in music, Tom, I don't forget.
Always so grateful for our friendship.

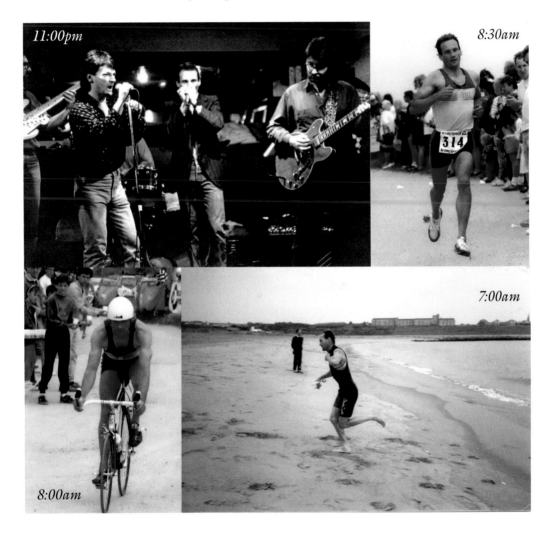

Music has always been such a huge part of my life. Several times gigs clashed with sporting competitions. I can remember competing in the North and South Tyneside triathlons where early starts were always the name of the game, 7:00am or thereabouts. I would play with the band on Saturday night from 9:00 to 11:30, travel home at midnight, be in bed by 1:00am, lie wide awake, get out of bed AT 5:00am and travel to the beach at either of the above and into the freezing North Sea before going on to winning those events.

Diet and Nutrition

Here's a brief preface to the subject which follows which is about **'Nutrition'** *and its immense influence on just about 'everything' a living person does or contemplates doing! So important is nutrition, it has the capacity to substantially extend your years and help keep you out of hospital, whilst additionally maintaining, or indeed improving, the all-important quality of your life, but conversely a poor choice can just as easily inhibit life's possibilities whilst also having the capacity to cut your life so drastically short! Furthermore, regardless of what some would have you believe, the subject need be neither complex nor difficult to understand nor is sensible eating and drinking expensive to employ!*

Have you ever watched on archive film, the workings of a steam-train, perhaps an engine similar to the iconic Flying Scotsman or the equally impressive Mallard? When I was a kid we lived within 20 metres of the busy East Coast main railway line, the one that runs between London's Kings Cross and Edinburgh's Waverley station, so close in fact was that five year old laddie to the line that often I would jump up from my bed (that I shared with my six year old sister Linda), in the middle of the dark night because I thought the train was about to come straight in through our bedroom window before leaving through the front door at the other side! Now next to our two up two down council house, and adjacent to the main line, was the 'bottom green', and on this hallowed turf we spent countless hours running, playing football and cricket, and as the trains sped past we'd occasionally pause from our energetic games for a few fleeting seconds as the train, engulfed in a dense cloud of coal induced smoke roared on to its destination. Apparently, a few years before I even kicked a ball on the green, the 'Scotsman' flew past on this very same line one day, the 30th November 1934, whilst in the process of creating a world record of 100mph for the 393 mile journey between the two capital cities. The train, at major expense, had clearly been set-up to perfection, not dissimilar perhaps to the 'Olympic athlete' as they also diligently prepare for the performance of a lifetime (also at major expense!). All *trials had been done and nothing had been left to chance. Only one thing left then, and that's the momentous act of **'fuelling'** the train as it powers along flat-out on its epic one-off 'perceived' record breaking journey! All the specialist expertise and the countless hours of preparation will be meaningless and futile if the energy needed to propel the machine onwards is not exact and 'spot-on' and up to the pluck and rigours of this majestic test! The train is powered by coal, and coal in this instance is the gold mine, the driver, the feeder and the life-line as well as the energiser. The fuel used on this special historic day is plentiful, in my neck of the woods coal is everywhere, and is dug deep underground by very special people, that's out-of-sight miners who work way down below the earth's crust. Once unearthed the coal is brought to the surface before being delivered to the train, at which point a 'very' fit and able engineer wearing totally unglamorous coal black and sweat soaked overalls takes over and speedily feeds the fires while clutching a greasy basic shovel. In my imagined world, I see both the miner and the engineer as anonymous heroes, fit, strong and able, and the basic 'fuel' they use together to power this work-of-art train will be the difference between success or failure, for there is often a fine dividing line between 'success', and the accompanying hoorays and handshakes and perceived 'failure' which is accompanied somewhat differently by tears and the consolatory pats on the back!*

*Now I'm not a coal miner, engineer, mechanic, scientist, stoker or inventor (I struggle with punctures for god's sake), I am though a life-long 'human athlete', who through years of isolated trying accompanied by much 'trial and error' have learned another skill(I use the term lightly) and that competence is about how the human body works, particularly perhaps in various sporting arenas, **and there are similarities between the phenomena that is the engine outlined above and the stunning piece of kit which is the human form.** I've argued throughout this publication that the human body is something 'very, very special' particularly and more so perhaps in the first 10 years of its life when it's new, that's before we've had the chance to ruin it, and after a few fleeting years basic health often begins its silent gradual descent resulting in so many self-inflicted illnesses or health related conditions which in turn emanate into so many self-imposed limitations.*

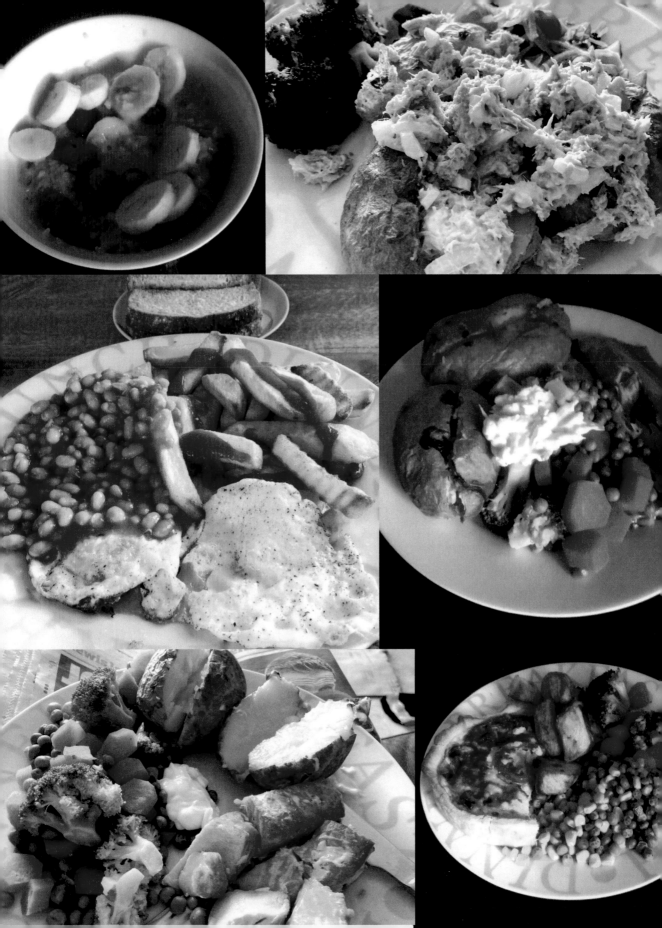

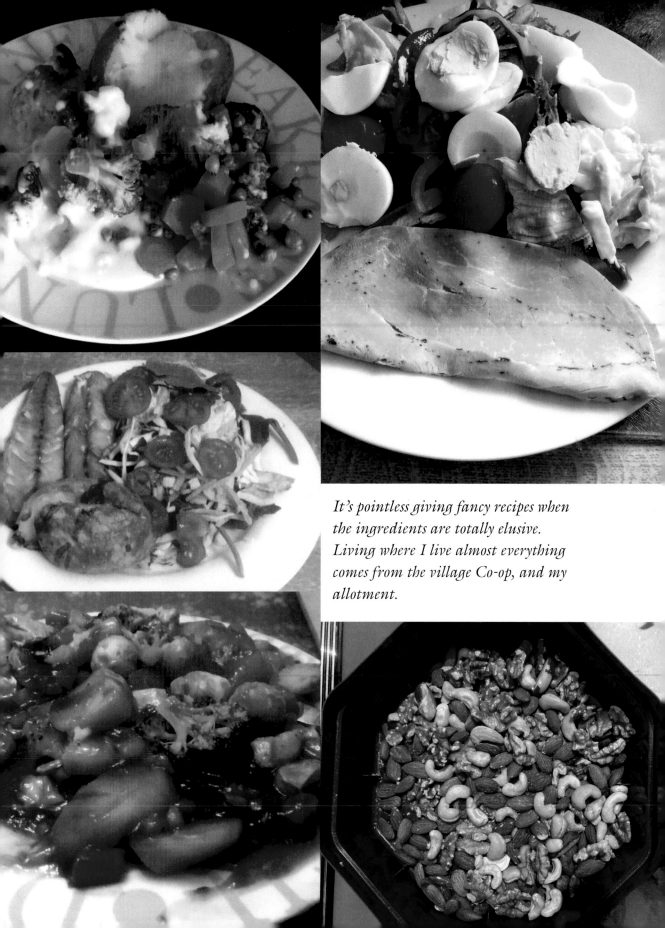

It's pointless giving fancy recipes when the ingredients are totally elusive. Living where I live almost everything comes from the village Co-op, and my allotment.

Feed and nourish the body with the same appetite and enthusiasm as the stoker feeds his train and for us life's possibilities abound, feed it with dregs, dross, waste and stale crumbs and just watch its demise! For most of us we are blessed with a choice, and as I've said elsewhere – the choice is ours to make, but in this instance choose very carefully!

Read on!

Some people believe that exercise alone is enough to ensure we remain healthy, WRONG! Indeed I'd go a stage further and say – some athletes aren't particularly healthy.

Exercise, amongst other things, creates a healthy, fit, efficient heart which, as mentioned previously, is best referred to as a 'pump'. The pump, however, is just one part of the system. The pipes which feed the system are of equal importance and physical exercise does little for the maintenance of the 'pipes'.

Exercise looks after the heart and NUTRITION looks after the blood vessels which feed the heart.

This subject, more than any other connected within the domain of health, drives me to distraction – there is so much total rubbish talked and portrayed in a never-ending stream of often complex, unpractical, expensive and debatable advice – aimed at whom? Currently (7/3/2021), and for many years, magazines and newspapers have 'saturated' their publishings with endless claims of 'miracle' life-saving nutritional information. Then running alongside the papers and magazines we are inundated with an abundance of 'cooking' programmes forever on our television screens with most of their offerings appearing to be in total contrast and incompatible with the 'healthy' advice the media advisory panels dish out (pun intended). The cooking programmes are about 'taste' and presentation, and seem to have the opposite philosophy of the *'eat well live forever'* health books. After all this I am left assuming Editors choose the inclusion of the countless page after page of colourful recipes, and health advice, simply because it is a cheap way of filling their pages, and doesn't the info all come from the labs anyhow, i.e. 'research, studies, and scientific experiments'! For every person who eats a boat load of apples and dies at 70, there are just as many who don't and go on to 90! Explain?

There is an never-ending growing number of people, presumably making a boat load of money, by advertising 'special' diets which consist of food and drink which have 'been around forever', lettuce, tomatoes, etc, etc, covered in a generous coating of olive oil, packaged with a mouth-watering label . Go walking, folks, eat and drink with some thought, laugh whenever you can, and most of the latter will cost you nothing. People aren't being good to you with their 'secrets' for nothing, you are paying their mortgages while at the same time ensuring the same newly promoted 'celeb' gets a seat on daytime telly programmes, keep it simple.

Forget exercise for a moment, and regardless of the above comments, I'm not in any way trivialising the subject of nutrition – far from it, because my view is that whatever you ingest in terms of eating and drinking, is very likely to have the greatest effect on both your current and long term health. Why is that? It's simple, it's because we all have to eat and drink if only to sustain life and wake up tomorrow, so we don't have an option, feel like it or not you will eat and drink; whereas with exercise there is an option, you choose to do it, or like most, you can easily avoid it – as you would a plague!

Can I just remind anyone reading any of this book that I do feel it necessary to occasionally repeat some chosen words from the book's title otherwise without words such as **'unique' and 'seventy year experiment'** this book will turn into 'just another' repetitive, and boring run of the mill book on a subject covered so many times by those with a certificate or two; in truth if I felt the latter was the case (just another book) I would never have started it.

So, here I am at 70 years of age, and at the moment, that's today, with 425 'consecutive' every day 'training' ('training', not to be confused with 'exercising') on a bike, swimming or running, and amounts of strength/mobility work thrown in, and much more recreational stuff besides. *Yesterday I did a time trial – 'flat out' (couldn't have tried much harder) – two hours of undulating cycling; I followed that up with 25 minutes' strength and core exercises, then dug my allotment for two hours (and walked the dog twice)* – now that is by my standards a 'typical', and fairly normal day. More to the point, I've 66 years of the same energy sapping life behind me. There's nothing unusual in the solitary term 'seventy years' of course, because I sit within an age category that consists of millions of us! However, I'm not sitting writing this with a shirt and tie on as most media writers present themselves; I am in fact sitting in t shirt and tracksuit bottoms. What is different is that my body has quite probably done what a bare 'miniscule' number of people on the planet has done – *from the exercise front I am an absolute 'oddment',* few can even begin to imagine the enormity of my athletic involvement over my current life span, and I've done it all so very quietly, I barely exist! Now take out the 'athletic' tag, and I have previously mentioned once or twice how, as a human being, I am the most 'ordinary' person you're ever likely to meet. I'm a heterosexual male of 'reasonable' intelligence (yes ok – debatable perhaps), with a family and have, like many, a few additional hobbies I fit in as time permits. Going back a while, I went to school and never missed a day (see chapter 'once upon a time'), then almost immediately joined the Royal Marines and was never laid up sick or injured; I then left after several years, with little other than the words 'an exemplary' and 'very professional Royal marine who should do well in the future', the latter written or attached within my brief discharge document. I was working (labouring – now wouldn't you just know it, ha!) within five days (I got lucky) and worked thereafter uninterrupted for approximately 35 years in the health and fitness industry, before my enforced retirement at 60 due to cutbacks. In all my life to date I was never sick, never had benefits and was never unemployed, *BUT always an athlete*! In fact, *'an athlete from birth right up to and including today'*. Now, please don't interpret the last few righteous sounding words as in any way boastful – the sentence and anything similar, are quite possibly the hardest statements I have ever written or likely to write and it unsettles me greatly to maybe come across as someone with a highly inflated arrogant view of himself, but if I am to have a view on this segment of this book I have to identify myself again, and reassuringly all the latter are fact!

So, let's have a look at diet and nutrition. **I can state with certainty that I have eaten the same 'Geordie' food my entire life, never changed, although it's fair to say I have 'sampled' other tasty morsels from time to time along the way. All my life I have used the same staple diet I eat today (potatoes with almost all my dinners) and that's because it tastes great and it appears, up till now at least, to work perfectly, and for the most part the exotic recipes I see every day in the Media are rarely on my plate or menu.** I would hastily add, based on my physical attainments, that if I were to die tomorrow my nutritional intake still worked exceedingly well, while consistently fuelling my energetic and ever hungry demanding body, and most certainly was not responsible for my demise or my ending. I am (unlike many, it seems), not obsessed with simply staying alive regardless of quality of life. The word 'longevity' in terms of selling health, is more common than sand at the beach, with additional words such as 'research has indicated' that eating this that or the other will extend your life by 18 months! How often have you read that? And how the hell do they know that, especially as there are so many variables involved in an individual's lifespan.

On reflection, the food and drink I ingest, was British and initially designed to nourish workers in the heavy industries of Coal Mining (pitmen), Ship Building, House building, and people physically working the land. To briefly sum up my food – well, it tastes 'superb', it was/is cheap, is easy enough to prepare and there was always plenty in terms of availability – that's because most of it came from local farms as well as back gardens and allotments and at other times if scarce then the local Co-op or travelling door-to-door greengrocers were the providers. At the moment, as I write, my family are still eating potatoes from my allotment which I planted a year ago, and in two weeks I'll be planting them again for another year. I've eaten potatoes all my life almost every day and currently I am informed by the 'Lab disciples' that they're carbohydrate, starch – bad for you! On a similar theme, so is rice, pasta, breakfast cereals and (surely not) bread too. Where's the proof? In a test tube on a bench? Bet a lot of the researchers are overweight. For seventy years I've eaten it, and won several hundred 'extreme' athletic events. My nutritional providers didn't used to talk in terms of a 'gram' here or a 'calorie' there, nor were they aware of the

'Mediterranean' diet which apparently makes you live forever! Those in the sun you see apparently don't die before a hundred and obviously never get ill! Worst job in the world? An Undertaker in the Mediterranean countries – because they're all on benefits or furlough – there's no business, you see, because they're all just too flaming healthy!

A lot of the talk today revolves around the importance of 'low' carbohydrate diets – well, once again my diet then and as it is now was/is immersed in extremely high amounts of carbohydrate. If I hadn't competed for GB in sport, then I could easily have represented my nation in eating. It is important to say, however, that my carbohydrate intake was mainly in the category of 'complex' Carbs, potatoes, wholemeal bread, cereals, fruit, vegetables and varieties of pasta dishes, as opposed to sweet confectionery products – although I have a sweet tooth as well.

Presumably the fuel used for an F1 car is measured by the car's performance; food for me is measured pretty much the same way – by performance. My daily non-complex nutrition has enabled me to perform with distinction for 70 years, I include infancy in the total! In my life, the men and women in the white overalls with the test tubes and the graphs never existed! No one handed me research and studies; I wouldn't have had time to read the data anyhow!

I hope that having written the earlier paragraphs of this chapter, that I haven't trivialised the importance of the nutrition subject, if so it wasn't intended, as mentioned in the opening lines as far as I'm concerned within the health subject there is nothing more important than our diet, and fortuitously eating and drinking is far easier than exercising because the latter entails going out in the wind, sun and rain every day – it's far easier to be lazy, sit still, watch telly and be merry. But be merry with a 'careful' eye on the tastes that make you merry.

Daily dietary requirements can be broken down into several individual sections, and basically we need some of each section to obtain a balanced healthy diet, that's a diet which provides us with the ingredients of energy, growth, repair and thermal insulation.

Carbohydrates (energy providing fuel)

In simple terms there are two types of carbohydrate; one is nutritionally sound, the other is of dubious content.

Complex carbohydrates

Complex carbohydrates consist of 'whole' foods (as portrayed in an advert – 'nowt teken out') such as wholemeal bread and wholegrain cereals, potatoes, brown rice, wholemeal pasta, fruit, nuts and vegetables, and high in liquid to keep us hydrated. These foods are high in slow burning energy, vitamins and minerals, fibre, and are low in fat, providing the servings aren't saturated in 'rich' sauces. Fibre is an essential ingredient which works the internal digestive system.

I once completed an Ironman triathlon (setting a new British record in the process). Now the event consists of a 2.4mile open water swim (in trunks those days), 112mile cycle stage again on a fairly basic 531 bike on 32 spoke GP4 wheels, without disc wheel or tri-bars, and finishing off with a marathon (26.2mile run). It took me 9hrs 37mins using basic equipment, so very different from that used these days. I mention the latter endurance event because it fits in well with the complex carbohydrate diet – slow burning fuel with naturally occurring vitamins and minerals – I used repeatedly in both the build-up and throughout the event. In training for the event my brother-in-law Duncan would drive me up to Edinburgh at five in the morning, at which point I'd cycle the 114 miles back home non-stop in a little over five hours (with two bananas and two water bottles) and immediately run for an hour off the bike; I'd then swim two miles in late afternoon (140 lengths). In offering up this information you can see the importance of your 'fuel' when taking on events of that nature. Longevity? I'm still here, little has changed, and I'm thriving!

On another occasion, I won the North Eastern Counties Marathon title on a hilly course from 250 athletes from all over the country in 2hrs 25m 26s. On that occasion I used something called the 'Carbo load diet', prior to the event, which briefly meant at six days beforehand I did a long run, about 18 miles, then ate only proteins and fats (no carbs) for three days, depleting my body of any carbohydrates, then thereafter and leading up to the race ate mainly complex carbs, filling up again, in the process topping up my storehouse the liver, muscles and blood stream with clean, easy to burn energy. I won by about two minutes and following a brief interview 'jogged' the mile or so back to the 'strip', had a shower, drove home and had a mountainous meal of the usual and an apple crumble pudding to follow. As mentioned, trial and error and personal 'experimentation'. I had no coach and no advisors, so when I talk about issues of this nature, I've been there and done it. My wife and sons ate whatever I was having only nowhere near as much; I'd eagerly watch the three of them, always ready to clean their plates as well if they left anything! I'm still 10st 3lbs and got all my own teeth except for two 'quitters!'

Simple Carbohydrates (I read a very sad article today 16/4/21, which identified how the misuse of certain drinks intended as 'health' products, can result in catastrophic organ failure when consumed in huge proportions. These drinks are not illegal and are common, easy to acquire products available all over the place, and when taken in extremes they can be life threatening. Too much sugar, in all its varying forms is not healthy – beware!!!)

In comparison to complex carbohydrate, simple carbohydrates, although providing an energy source, are far less nutritionally rich. Foods that fit within this category are confectionary products such as sweets, chocolate (especially white – no offence!), cakes, biscuits etc. There are few if any vits/minerals in these and they are short of fibre, the energy burn is quick, additionally they can be high in hidden fat, leading to more calories to hump around.

Here's an interesting thing. The Ironman I competed in had feed stations at various distances; however, the tables were lacking what many of us needed and the chopped bananas had dried out in the sun. There were boiled sweets though, but try running with gob-stoppers clanking against your teeth after nine hours of physical labour. There was also pickled gherkins, I'm serious (the organisers clearly had a bizarre sense of humour). Finally, there were also copious amounts of de-fizzed coca cola in open cups, the latter were for me at least a 'life-saver' honestly. When you are 'empty' and operating on nothing other than mental grit and 'muscle memory', the coke gave an immediate spontaneous lift that was heaven-sent. The feed stations during the latter stages of the last discipline marathon were every 1km on these forest tracks; my intake of coke would propel me onwards with the ingredients of sugar, dubious liquid and the drug like caffeine for approximately 800 metres till I was empty again; consequently I'd labour on for the final 200 metres before receiving another fix – this went on till the finish. The sugar in the black stuff may well be responsible for my two missing back teeth! Oh well, you win some and you lose some, eh?

Protein (body building and repair)

There is some form of protein in most foods. However, the main sources of protein are found in meat, fish, eggs and dairy produce, milk etc. Some nutritionists recommend high protein diets; however, many products which are high in protein tend to be high in fats as well, so be careful. Muscle is built and repaired on protein, so it sits firmly within a balanced diet, as always balance is the key.

Fat

An amount of fat is a necessity within our diet to provide insulation from the cold; it also helps protect our vital organs, and fat allows fat soluble vitamins to do their work; furthermore fat can be used as an energy source, particularly for endurance sports – once carbs/sugars have been utilised within the muscles, liver and bloodstream then fat becomes the next available energy source, hence it is rare to see a fat marathon runner or Tour-de-France cyclist. A negative with fat as an energy source is that apparently it takes greater degrees of oxygen to convert it to fuel. Having said some positives regarding fat, nutritionists warn us regularly about the negatives of harbouring too much, which will lead to unhealthy weight gain, and fur-up blood vessels which in turn reduces blood flow, and remember, as discussed, blood transfers essential energy and oxygen around the body. The smaller the blood vessels in terms of circumference (due to the furring up of the walls) the more susceptible we become to the trapping of a blood clot (cutting off the blood supply) which may lead to a heart attack.

There are two types of fats found in our diet, one to be watched closely as too much is a potential foe. So, we have **saturated fats** often found in red meats, sausages, burgers, bacon and gammon, as well as hard cheeses, cream cakes and fry-ups. Polyunsaturated (often referred to as **unsaturated fat)** found in fish oils and vegetable such as sunflower or corn are healthier, nuts are currently believed to be a very healthy choice, not just for 'good fats' but for other sound nutritional needs.

Vitamins and Minerals

There are two types of vitamins; these are water soluble, and fat soluble, meaning that differing vitamins work within each – water and fat. Water soluble vitamins as the name suggests work within liquid, so we can't store them in the body because we secrete them in sweat, the breathing process and when using the toilet. So, we need a constant supply. Vitamin C, and the B group are two of the best known and are generally found in complex carbohydrates such as fruit and vegetables; also if you don't have much in the way of fruit and veg, then a tablet form is harmless enough because any excess will be naturally secreted, so you end up with highly expensive urine!!

A quick word on FRUIT. All my life I've eaten a mountain of fruit. I have a sweet tooth and the fructose (sugar in fruit) found in fruit fortunately satisfies that urge for sweetness. As an athlete and a lifestyle immersed in physical work, I have spent my life sweating, and the purpose of sweat is to cool the body down when it exceeds a certain temperature. Sweat is liquid and when the body's liquid content is low its ability to physically work is hindered, reducing levels of performance. As sweat leaves the inner body it takes with it water-soluble vitamins and minerals. Replacing these minute substances is essential, and fruit in all its varying forms is saturated with water-soluble vitamins and minerals (depending on the type of fruit). Up to 90% of fruit is liquid, hence it's all very health-promoting. The good news is fruit is all relatively cheap, is readily available – there is little if any time required for preparation, straight from the bag and into your gob! One last thing on fruit, it is best eaten alone and on an empty stomach, so breakfast time is ideal – even after sleep you may be dehydrated. If you eat fruit with other foods, it delays the process of digestion – a bit like putting your best shirt in the washer with your overalls…they all get tangled up. So you wash them separately! Eating fruit between meals is also snacking healthily. One more thing, don't rely on thirst as your activator to drink. A better guide is to check your urine and a clear colour is best.

A balance. I can recall having a discussion some time ago with a work colleague who was about to take part in a testing endurance event in the Cheviot hills of Northumberland, and he mentioned the weather forecast for his event was going to be unusually very hot. As such he was drinking copious amounts during the build-up to ensure he would be totally 'hydrated' before the event! Until, that is, I mentioned that he was probably swilling huge amounts of water soluble vitamins and minerals through his system which may well result in cramp. The point I was making, and still would, is that too much of almost anything will create abnormal reactions, now that's just common sense!

Medication. When the pandemic occurred about a year ago with a touch of altruism I immediately delivered a letter to my local clinic volunteering to deliver prescriptions around my local community to those less able and therefore struggling to collect their own medication; to be honest it makes me feel good to help a little. Now I don't know if this routine is universal, but where I live the Doctors won't allow you (even now a full year later, and there's only 47 Covid cases in the whole of Northumbria) into the clinic in case you are a 'virus carrier' who might hand it to them, you see, and you're just not worth the risk; so when I go to collect the prescriptions I have to join a queue outside the clinic and only when I get to the front am I allowed to enter the building. Hands scrubbed clean for at least 20 seconds and with my Lone Ranger mask tightly applied, one in one out, is the strict policy! In the process of going to the clinic every week it's suddenly hit me how many people are on pill-type medication – there is nearly always a queue, and I'm only up there a tiny fraction of the time. So the taking of pills is a 'huge' community pastime!

Artie Blues Boy White (amid some beautiful guitar playing) sings 'Doctor Doctor what's wrong with me, I need a pill to wake me up another to make me sleep, another to make me drink and another to make me stop, a pill for my top and one for my bottom!' etc.

Pills – Come on, tell me it's an expensive joke.

As a working amateur athlete I was, and remain, very frugal. My mantra always was and still is 'keep it simple', don't go looking for something that doesn't exist, I'm talking in terms of 'miracle' options in training, equipment and even nutritional products. If you find 'something' that you believe gives you the edge on your fellow competitors it's probably illegal (illegal is not a sick bird by the way) anyhow. If what follows had been in a Monty Python script, we'd be howling!

In our daily newspaper today, there is a full page (and presumably at the perceived expense it's worth their while) advertising 40 tubs of different supplement pills, all it seems (I'm guessing the adverts don't actually state it) have certain unique wonderful properties which will, I assume, heal, improve, prevent, assist or maybe delay some sort of an expected onset of something nasty. The most expensive pills are reduced from £45.99 to £27.59. Descriptions are severely limited if available at all. Here's a couple though: 'We've *combined the highest grade Hyaluronic Acid with Green Lipped Mussel Extract to create this new formula'.* Or – *'Evening Primrose Oil is rich in a substance called Gamma Linolenic Acid (GLA').* Last one – *'Acidophilus – Contains around 50 million Lactobacillus Acidophilus 'friendly bacteria' per capsule* (wonder how they keep all the little bacteria in there, 50 million, man?). I don't care how 'friendly' they are, that's a lot of bacteria to be swilling down with your Earl Grey, your best

Nescafe or your Guinness. In the same paper same day there's a celeb kind of celebrating their health, apart from the self-confessed use of Botox, Fillers – (wonder what they are?), and facelifts, the individual also takes 30 supplement tablets every day and has been apparently for the past 45 years – I could be wrong, nevertheless my mobile says that's 283,500 pills! Wonder if their partner knows? Wonder if their partner occasionally comments: 'You ok, pet? You're looking a bit peaky, maybe you need a pill, a pick-me-up or two!'

Now a lot of us work on the basis that with all things health orientated 'more is better'; mind you, on a personal basis I'm not suggesting or advocating the latter. Nevertheless it's got me wondering, what would happen to me if every day I took one pill from each of the aforementioned advertised 40 tubs, I mean logically speaking if they are all so different while being full of some sort of 'goodness' with very encouraging health-related substances inside their shiny coloured shell, then that being the case, on 'just' 40 tablets a day, would I be able to ride my bike faster and for longer, or would I be down to four minute miles, or perhaps be able to swim the channel (I'd expect there and back at those prices), or would Jennifer be frantically running away from me whilst screaming ' for god's sake, not again, Mick – I'll get the police, mind!' After all, at 'one a day from each tub', that's 40 a day, times by 7 isn't that 280 tablets a week? Add on your egg and chips and that's a lot of presumed goodness!

As mentioned elsewhere, and bearing in mind I'm seventy and counting, I have occasionally over the years tried one or two of the more well-known supplement pills, I'm talking Vitamin C, the B group (both water soluble), or Cod Liver Oil for my joints, I've used little else; regardless, I really never noticed any change, good, bad, or indifferent, so pretty quickly I gave up and went back to my jam sandwiches, big stodgy home-made family meals, fruit and nuts, and porridge. It seems to me that as human beings we are all so very receptive to outside influences, we can be persuaded by the better or more proficient salespeople to buy just about anything, especially if the positivity is present during the sale; I mean, we can be gullible, can't we? For years I have been aware of something referred to as the **placebo** effect. The whole issue revolves around *'beliefs', that's self-belief or implanted beliefs!* **Have a look at this:**

Placebo!

I read a book lately by a guy from Whitley Bay called Tappy Wright. Now Tappy has since died but before he went he led a very interesting life as a rock group Road Manager – he looked after The Animals for years as well as Jimi Hendrix, Ike and Tina Turner and many more. Anyhow, at one point in the book he relates a story whereby his boss asked him to drive up to Newcastle (from London) in the middle of the night, pick up a very important package and return with it immediately back to London. Now Tappy wasn't too pleased – as mentioned it was the middle of the night and he was already tired out! Anyhow before he left he grumbled a bit in Eric Burdon's company at which point Eric said words to the effect of 'here, Tappy, take one of these, it'll help you out' before handing him a small pink pill. Fully believing there was something special in the pill (known then I think as an 'upper') Tappy begrudgingly swallowed it before setting off for the Toon. The effect was instantaneous: he was wide awake, singing loudly and a bundle of energy. He picked up the package and returned forthwith back to the capitol. Seeing Eric the next morning he said something like 'Hey, Eric, what the hell was in that pill, it was amazing?' Eric, laughingly replied – 'Oh that, Tappy, it was nothing other than a woman's contraceptive pill!'

Now I am a difficult person to sell anything to (I'm not only talking goods), I need proof of most things before I even contemplate a purchase, but I have to say I do believe in the philosophy attached to placebos, there has been so many believable examples of similar instances. Some might just palm it off as 'positive talk' (so often used by sports psychologists) and positive talk may help instil positive beliefs, and they may have a point, nevertheless being positive and even having positive mantras are a real bonus, whether it be in fitness or nutrition! I always put my right shoe on first (nobody knows that) and I'm still here!!! So why would I want to change 'a winning formula'?

Going back to today's newspaper advert I started this chapter with, and discussed above, the 'sales pitch' has got to be taken on trust, because none of us ordinary punters are in a position to contradict (apart from my occasional aggravating negativity), nor are we in a position to extol the virtues of products we've never seen before, let alone tried, so we work at best on a positive assumption.

Regardless, if the wording is convincing (and these companies are pros), likewise if the visual display is eye catching and the price is ok (remember this is a *sale* with big reductions, which we're told won't last!), or you are desperate enough, and the ingredients (you've never heard of) have a miracle element somehow attached to the 'tub' – well, why not give them a go! As well as the above, there are just hundreds of products which apparently self-heal – and without the need to queue up outside at the current 'empty' clinic or to travel to outpatients and annoy – but there is a monetary price to pay of course!!

With all these miracle products, I wonder? Do we need a *National Health Service*?

Another current update: Fresh from the printers and into today's newspaper the smiling ever so healthy face comments. Magic copper insoles stopped my knee pain; No more foot pain and I've lot ten pounds; I am now able to walk pain free; Tiredness, fatigue, ill health were all getting worse until I found ...'And this one is a first for me – 'Brain Fog' is a by-product of the pandemic, so try bullet proof brain octane, or prime fifty and cognition capsules... As well as other brain capsules cheap at the price of £80.95' and so it goes on. Some products as you'd expect are endorsed by celebrities (and they should know, eh?!) and all are accompanied by photos of the happiest smiling people you're ever likely to meet! Some other health tips in yesterday's paper include 'recent research' shows that a 50 minute run 'just once a week' will help you live longer; the thing is how many of us can actually run for 50 minutes? Additionally, how long would it take for most of us to reach that 50 minute standard? Another article says that to prevent falls try balancing on one leg at least once a day – apparently to do so is also an important test of your 'brain health' – beats taking the 11 plus exam I guess, I'd be top of the class and straight into Oxford or Cambridge! Another advocates skipping to improve bone health, now there is some credence in that simply because bone strength is improved or maintained by regular physical 'impact' activities, but surely walking is less complex for at least 99% of the population? Besides, let's be realistic, how many of us can skip, and more to the point how many of us are prepared to skip regularly if we aren't prepared to walk? LONGEVITY is the key to almost everything; short fixes rarely work, except maybe for the use of a firing squad I suppose, and that's a bit extreme. Another said, you could also try 'standing up' to eat because it helps reduce how much you eat because your food apparently tastes worse than it does when seated, so we may be putting off asking for seconds! Drumming (as in musical instruments) eases mental pressure and helps ward off viruses such as flu, and so streets full of drum kits of the Keith Moon or John Bonham type are the noisy future, eh? At the same time 'shout' yourself fitter – it boosts oxygen intake!! Where did the term 'love thy neighbour' come from? More to the point when did it die out – 'following a newspaper article in the year 2021 – that's when!

AND ANOTHER THING!

Weight loss (worth a mention)

'If you put too much fuel in a fuel tank it'll spill right over the top with the excessive waste materialising down the side of the car; now if you put too much fuel in your gob and allow the overflow to transfer to your ever receptive gut (it has to go somewhere) – in a short while the surplus will also materialise, same place, down your sides, onto your butt, and around your stomach. How do you prevent this? Don't keep filling the tank up; or, if you do, make sure you burn some of it off, before you top it up again! Come on, you know that, don't you, of course you do. Now once again I'm not telling you what to do, wouldn't dream of it, and I've no right to do that; but your body is your responsibility, whatever you do – it's 'your choice', but if you get fat or ill, don't blame the NHS! It's got nothing to do with them; it wasn't their choice or fault, was it?

Without a doubt it's one of the most debated subjects in the western world, even very fit people become obsessed and even depressed about their weight. Losing weight can clearly be very simple for some and yet immensely difficult for others, genetics and the speed or rate of metabolism can play a major role, and we differ, some are lucky, others not so, but, and it's been said forever – we often make our own luck.

Essentially if we exercise regularly and then don't replace all the calories we've expended then we should be able to lose weight. The exception may be that as we become leaner we may well also become heavier because we have increased muscle mass and muscle weighs more than fat.

There is a view which says you can't be overweight and be healthy, but I beg to differ. My own view is that it is possible to be carrying a bit extra but be very fit with it. So, if your diet is nutritionally sound and you are exercising regularly, I'd say be wary but don't be overly concerned, enjoy your life but be vigilant, your body is 'phenomenal' – look after it with the same care and attention you give to your children and grandchildren.

WHO are you kidding!!!

A common occurrence in any gymnasium is for people to weigh themselves immediately after the workout. The information given at this time is misleading because your weight loss is due to liquid loss rather than fat loss. Don't get obsessed with weighing yourself every few hours, the best time is either in the morning when you get out of bed, or before your workout.

DIET NUTRITION – CONCLUSION!

The subject of nutrition is vast, just look at the market, so many pages of adverts in the press, many extolling 'miracle' properties; for most of us though the subject is relatively simple unless you have special requirements possibly due to illness so I'll leave the subject there. I have personally experimented with legal nutritional products when I could be bothered – that's the truth. Some additional vitamins such as the water soluble Vitamin C and some everyday minerals, I can honestly say that despite my unusual energetic life I never found anything that was an 'obviously' beneficial bonus. That may be because my daily diet has been very good and everything I needed for 25 hour training weeks and more were already boiling in the pans and pots! I eat loads of fruit, fortunately

I like it, and as already identified my meals were/are mundanely basic, potatoes, porridge, bread, vegetables, nuts (I like them too) as well as tea and coffee. As far as food goes if there is plenty of it I'll smile, in contrast if I go for what I'd call an 'expensive' meal (above £7.50) and I have to make a cheese sandwich when I get home I grimace and curse! But I also accept in this regard (going for a meal) 'god knows I'm boring!' I'd sooner go to the chippy!

I read a statement a long while ago which captures the thinking on food 'consumption'. It read, 'do you like to eat a lot? Want to learn how to eat a lot?' Here it is: 'eat a little, that way you'll be around long enough to eat a lot!'

There is a huge amount of that dreaded word 'research' around which says amongst other things, 'if you want to increase an animal's lifespan, cut down on the amount of food it eats'. Now we all know that consuming food and drink is a pleasurable pastime, in fact it is so pleasurable that often the more we get the more we want. Why? Basically because, as I've stated elsewhere, the body will accustom itself to whatever we throw at it. Whether it be physical fitness orientated or nutrition orientated, if we persist along the right guidelines sooner rather than later we change.

Back to EXERCISE. Pre-event, during, and after the event nutrition (once again I was bucking the trend).

Remember when I talk health and fitness, my trump card is 'the vast majority of my findings are based on what I've done, how I've done it, and what the results were, not what others have done and how they may have done it'! I wasn't coached or tutored, I didn't copy, I couldn't, I was a working amateur, 37/40 hour working weeks, never unemployed, never sick and with a family to provide for, as such I lived my life **'probably like you'**, on a very real monetary budget, what I had financially, was in my pocket so to speak, I never knew, and still don't, what 'social monetary benefits' were/are, and that if nothing else is a simple non-complex way to live your life. In many ways I'd learned from my elders and went on to copy (at least in principle) the routines of people in the 1950s. There were little piles of money which were ever present on top of sideboards or mantelpieces, rent money, coal, insurance, milk, school dinners and hire purchase agreements, if there was anything left we might be lucky and get a three-penny piece once or in an exceptional week even twice a week, and we smiled!

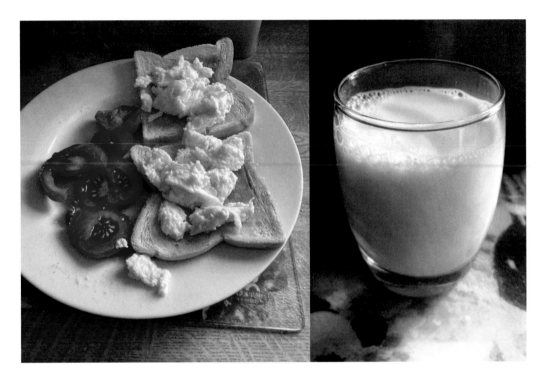

After exercise, protein, carbohydrate, and liquid, and all cheap as chips.

My sporting equipment by comparison to so many others was ordinary, it's still the same. **When I was winning cycle races between 50 and 61 years of age, my bike occasionally became a magnet, others would gather around and look at it, pick it up to assess its weight, feel the tyre pressures, and study the gear ratios, as I quietly stood grinning, just amused. Following their examinations I would occasionally have someone enquire further with 'is this yours, Mike?'** Maybe it was the stabilisers? The questions and analysis wasn't ridicule, all my fellow competitors were lovely people*, I had no enemies, their interest was based purely on intrigue and genuine curiosity, mainly, I assume, because other riders had much more eye catching kit. I'm racing this Wednesday (12/5/2021) and nothing will have changed, I'll still use the same bikes I had 20 years ago. For most of my years of racing bikes either in Triathlons, Time Trials or occasional Road Races, my racing bike frames were 531/753/853 Steel frames, with decent chain sets etc – but by no means the best. My NPCC skinsuits were based on a 'sized estimate', and didn't wash well, in fact they would have hung better on my wife Jennifer (no offence, pet!); arguably they may even have appeared like I borrowed them, a little like putting newspapers in your shoes when a kid (to make 'em fit) but thankfully while in the saddle the size discrepancy wasn't too obvious – even if they were a 'bit big'! On hindsight some riders probably couldn't pass me for laughing – I'm exaggerating – I hope.

*When talking about my fellow competitors, I always found it strange that very few, when asked how they were, would say *'great, I'm in good shape'*, most either hedged their bets and shrugged or more commonly murmured totally negative comments such as *'oh I've been up all night with the bairn, I'll not go well today'* or reply *'I'm not fit, too busy at work to get the miles in'*. Or maybe the old favourite, *'I've got a stinking cold'*, with perhaps an ambiguous *'oh don't ask!!'* comment. They'd then proceed to ride like Mr Wiggins. Strange! In contrast, when I was asked, often by the event's timekeepers at the start as you waited anxiously for the countdown having freewheeled up to the line, I always made a point of being very positive – *'terrific'* I'd say, *'very fit, very healthy'* and they'd reply with a grin *'no change there then, you always are'*. My philosophy was that I had absolutely nothing to gain by mumbling untrue negatives, and you know what – no one was bothered about me (or you) anyhow, the questions were just basic human etiquette, niceties, none of us were that important, well perhaps only to ourselves whilst dwelling within our own selfish little worlds.

Although my main aim when writing my five books (two were work related) was first and foremost to be original and different otherwise there was no point, nevertheless you can't escape factual info based, for example, on issues such as 'carved in stone' principles such as interval training, or what do complex carbohydrates do for you etc. and although included in this book (because you can't avoid them when writing on health or fitness) you can read about those subjects and many more from literally hundreds of books so I haven't written in major detail – because it's been done before. But I was the best Triathlete in the country for a few years winning many British Championships, and before that I was racing and winning marathons, before that I represented the Marines in four different sports and at my boarding school in the hills, I did 'everything' – rugby, cricket, football, athletics, cross country and gymnastics – and when all that was over I went on to win almost 80 cycle races, and when my contemporaries had long since retired from sporting competitions I was finishing 2nd in Park Runs, at 65 (at one event I was 11th from 557 finishers and I was touching 69) and 12th in outdoor Triathlons at 68, even winning a duathlon at 67. And yet apart from school and in the mob at this moment as I look back, I was somehow 'always old' ha ha, but it's true, on reflection that was probably because my youth was spent (straight from my boarding school at Bellingham), as a fighting soldier in the Royal Marines, so when I came out, well – I had some catching up to do. My trump card, on reflection, was that when I went into triathlon*, although in my 30s at the time, I'd already done an immense 'apprenticeship' and from running with Morpeth knew how to train and more importantly knew how to suffer. I had the heart and respiratory system of Tarzan and the physique of a 'middle weight' pro boxer. My main opponents, although ten years my junior, well they were still learning. I was British Champion when I was 37 and British Grand Prix Champion the same wonderful year, and the kids were still keeping me up all night and my bosses at work liked me because I was reliable, never sick and knew my job inside out!!

*My entry into the world of Triathlon came by chance one fine day in the staffroom at Ashington Leisure Centre. Leafing casually through a newspaper I came across an article (it's in front of me as I write, from 1982 I think) titled Looking for the Ironman. The headline was accompanied by Daley Thompson and a couple of others lying around on their backs on an athletics track having just completed the final event of a Decathlon (1,500 metres). It reads; *The ultimate athletic challenge is now on the starting blocks ready to arrive in Britain, America's current craze for pushing the body to the limit of its endurance has reached a gruelling climax in the triathlon – a torturous course of swimming, cycling and marathon running.* Brendan Foster was tasked by Nike to look at its possibilities over here, and apparently he'd had *'a great deal* *of interest, and* (I write as it reads) *people are not pooh-poohing the idea, it is not mad and* is **the ultimate test of fitness**. He went on to say *'it is likely to appeal to men of the SAS – I wouldn't take part,'* he said, *'I can't ride a bike!'*

Intrigued, within a day or two I went into the pool swam a mile front crawl, which was 72 lengths I think, an absolute doddle, and sent off to the recently formed British Triathlon Association and awaited their response. I was North Eastern Counties Marathon Champion at the time, could, I believed, swim like a fish, and all I needed was a bike – I bought (a big black one!) one from Ray Wears back street shop for £212 and the rest as they say is history!!!

A week in February 1986!

I set a new British Ironman record in Sweden later that year 1986, and for years I found my time embarrassing at 9hrs 37min, that is by comparison to what they are doing now. However, looking back now *I am really very proud of that performance and truly amazed it was that fast.* The journey with a GB team manager was done over two days by two trains, car, ferry, and then 'umpteen hours' over Europe while sitting in the back seat of his car to get to the event. Upon arriving, I was put up in a 'hut' beside the lake which was very nice, but in Sweden at that time of the year it never got dark, so sleeping, always my nemesis anyhow, was out of the question, so I probably hadn't slept for three days before the event. During the event, I swam the 2.4 miles in the 'cool' lake 'without' the now customary wetsuit, then rode the 112 undulating miles on a 531 steel-framed bike using 32 spoke GP4 wheels with heavy invulnerable tubular tyres and no tri-bars, no disc, and finished off with the 26.2mile marathon drinking de-fizzed coca cola (it was either that or 'dusty' water) to keep me going! Following the event, the next day we travelled the same way as we had arrived for two very uncomfortable days to get home *and I went back to work!!!* On reflection a lot of my life as an amateur athlete was very similar.

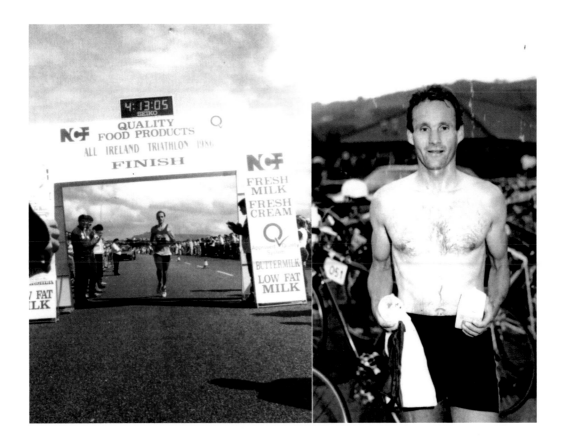

Sometimes when idling away the hours at home I'll pick up at random an old training diary (I've 45 or more kicking around) just to see what I was doing at 'today's' corresponding time 10, 20, 30 or 40 years ago, while also checking out the weather that day to see what the comparison was then. In front of me at this moment is a week in February 1986; at the time I was working at Ashington Leisure Centre, working an early and late shift. 10th Feb: am biked to work 17 miles, followed by swim 2000yards, Lunch time run 1hour, pm bike home 2 hours (good effort) pm swim 2000yards. Under reminders at the top of the page it reads: **A typical day's meals 12/2/86 –am porridge, 2 slices toast, tea, also – am apple, orange, pear, 4 slices bread, whole fruit jam, then for dinner 3 baked potatoes, few nuts, dates, apple, pm soup and 5 slices of bread, followed by boiled potatoes, fish, peas, tea and biscuits, supper porridge with raisins, followed by 3 slices of bread and jam, tea and an apple!! I WAS 10ST 3LBS and it seems always hungry – wonder why?**

Later in the year I was given an all-expenses paid invitation (with Jennifer) to compete in Sligo, Republic of Ireland in the 'All Ireland Triathlon Championships' (a half Ironman event). Similar to the above, the journey was arduous – we drove and 'sailed' to get there, travelled through the very dark night in our little red Beetle, and were stopped several times on the Northern Ireland side, by 'squaddies' with their rifles who searched our car and bags meticulously, before sending us on our way. As I remember it was a freezing cold sea swim, again no wetsuit, and from several hundred competitors I was second to Gerard Hartman (later to become Paula Radcliffe's physio) who was well behind me in the Europeans in Denmark in 1985 where I finished 8th and got the Bronze team medals with Glen Cook 5th and Pete Moysey 29th.

Talking about Ireland. Around about this time '85/86', Northern Ireland hosted the European short course relays; all transitions were guarded by squaddies, again with all the weapons, a bit 'eerie'; but what I remember most about that trip was going over the grimy sea with the team resplendent in our Great Britain tracksuits and reading the headline on the back page of a newspaper 'ALL GREAT BRITAIN SPORTING TEAMS A LEGITIMATE TARGET FOR IRA'!!!! Ha and here we were puking up in the rough water waiting to be shot – and guess who was a former Royal Marine Commando? By the way, on both those occasions in both sides of the Irish border, the events were first class, so warm and friendly, and my dealings with them both in the forces and at other times were always great, most are good people, warm, humorous and exceedingly helpful. Some may have read my adventures with Paddy Green in my autobiographies, now I'm smilling!!

European Triathlon (mixed) Relay Championships were at Mansfield on 27April 1986, and myself with Glen Cook, Sarah Coope, Howard Jones (the three had recently returned 'bronzed' from wintering in California) picked up the Silver Medals; it was either Holland or Germany who took gold I think. My personal three disciplines of the event began with an 11-mile run, followed by a 22-mile bike and an 880yrd swim. The legs were all different allowing each four-person team to decide who would compete in each section; running still being seen as my 'strength' I was delegated the longest run leg!

Now I've touched on this subject before but it may be interesting to some so I'll mention it again.

Competition food and drink.

I have never spent money on fancy food or drink (apart from Guinness). No bonny coloured energy bars and seldom on fashionable coloured miracle drinks. For events over two hours, I used 50% orange juice (concentrated carton type) mixed with 50% tap water; events over three hours the same thing but maybe with the addition of a banana or two and just a tiny snip of table salt in the bottle, depending on the weather. Two or three days before a big Triathlon or Marathon I carbo loaded on complex carbohydrate, meals made by Jennifer, and in between them I'd eat things like home-made scones and rock buns*. If I had a cycling competition such as a mid-week Time Trial in the evening after work, I would often have a tin of vegetable or tomato soup and two slices of bread and a cup of tea, that would be about two hours before the start. I'd have a shower and brush my teeth because it made me feel fresh and awake. Then I'd 'sip' tap water (supplied by Northumbrian Water, not the Co-op) up to the start. Occasionally if the weather was cold I'd have a small comforting coffee before I left my car for a 30minute warm-up spin, I don't take sugar. After the event or following intensive training *I'd drink milk*, and occasionally have a small glass of the same before bed, bit of protein and of course the liquid helped keep me hydrated overnight. My body weight gave me a lot of simple detail in a few seconds – if I was overweight slightly that was a good sign, if I was underweight (even by a pound or two) – it was a concern because I figured it was probably water I was short of not fat! Before big events, on the mornings, I didn't weigh myself at all, I wanted 'positives', not possible mental negatives – too late, best not know about any negatives at that stage. In the Ultra fit competition I mentioned earlier, I was underweight in the morning before the five-hour drive down, and when I arrived my urine was not its usual clear colour, trying to drink to remedy it was just too late, and on a very warm day in a humid hangar I'd messed up. The event was always going to hurt, but it hurt more than it needed to because I'd switched off; afterwards I was very dehydrated, felt weak and worse than anything I was so annoyed that I could allow that to happen. Amazing really when you think about it, so many athletes are so disciplined regarding their training, yet are prepared to sacrifice all that hard work by being so clumsy with their fuel. Have a 'holistic' view to everything, leave nothing to chance.

When coaching Daniel Dixon I'd enquire quite regularly as to whether he was cutting his toe nails or regularly cleaning his teeth, sure he felt there was something wrong with me, then I'd say you don't want feet problems or toothache in the Olympic final – now do you?

Milk *was my first consideration after a hard session – cheap as chips, protein, vitamins and minerals and of course all immersed in liquid to help hydrate me after the effort!*

*Rock Buns. I mentioned this before in my second autobiography.

In 1985 I travelled down to Milton Keynes for the British Triathlon Championships with a good friend of mine from Durham called Steve Brown; Steve was a smashing bloke and a very able triathlete. Anyhow when we arrived at our pre-arranged digs the night before the event, I sat on a bed, and took out my bate from a brown paper bag for a snack, and produced three or four of Jennifer's freshly baked 'rock buns'. Steve was watching me very closely primarily because as the current champion I was the favourite for another championship win. Anyhow Steve said, *'What you got there then, Mike?'* and I replied, *'Oh just rock buns, Steve, you want one?'* Steve momentarily hesitated, then staring at the raisin-speckled uneven bun replied, tongue in cheek *'oh yes please'*, followed by *'that's your secret eh, rock buns!'*

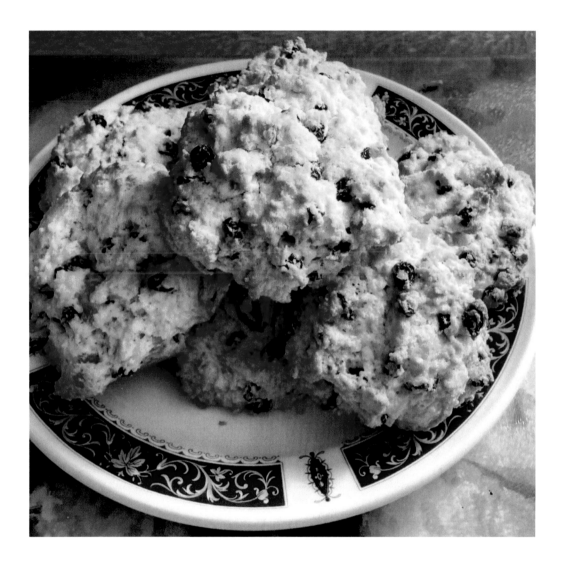

Anyhow to cut the story short, the next day the two of us stood eagerly by the vast Willen Lake, with another 400-plus adrenalin-soaked triathletes. Some two hours later I came round the final bend on the run, sprinted only to lose my title by three seconds. Later on in the day, the two of us travelled the lengthy journey back to Steve's house on the outskirts of Durham where my old banger was sitting on his drive. As we got out of the car Steve's wife and mother-in-law met us on the drive with an enthusiastic *'well, how'd you do?'.* 'Well,' said Steve, *'Mike was an unlucky 2nd, and I was 57th!' He* followed that up immediately with a pleading *'do you know how to make rock buns?'* as his bemused wife looked confusingly on. Steve was apparently captivated by the prospect of big inroads in his triathlon future as a result of the special nutritious 'secret'! ME? Well I should have eaten all four and as a result been able to sprint just that wee bit faster for the gold!

I've said this before but with something as important as this, I'll say it again. Your diet, short and long term, will have more effect on not only your current general daily health but also on your actual longevity on this planet of ours, and I'm talking 'HEALTHY life-span' here. My belief, and it's only me (and most certainly I'm not a prophet sent from above), is that of all issues connected in some way to our personal health – and that includes exercise – your consumption of the food and drink you choose will ultimately decide your very future and everything you do, so be very careful, my friends and eat well, because nutrition is a huge influence on just about everything you do or more to the point what 'you'd like to do!' perhaps a bit later!

For most of us, our state of health is nothing other than a consequence of choice. What we have is probably what we've chosen – CHOOSE CAREFULLY!

To Jennnifer, the best cook in the world, thank you. It says it all. All diet and nutrition photographs in this publication were home made by my wife followed by a quick mobile photograph.

Mental Health!!!

I started writing a 'little bit' on this subject because it is so very high profile and it has somehow turned into an extended and unintended essay, which includes an additional bit of history to compare the past with the current!

The best blues guitarist in the world, a certain Mr Buddy Guy, once said, 'If all I ever listened to was Count Basie, I'd only ever play jazz!' You'll see the link between Buddy's comment and what follows.

I don't believe people are born unhappy, we develop in all things as we go through life and are continually changing in views and thought, and that's because we are always open to influence is what I am saying. Have you ever subconsciously taken a tune or a musical rhyme to bed? The riff or the rhyme won't leave you alone as you try to find respite and sleep and you silently repeat the musical mantra and the more you repeat it the more engrained in our mind it becomes. Now, sit someone in a room for 24 hours a day, seven days a week and show them, and tell them, little other than morbidity, gloom and doom, sombre news, together with heartache accompanied by gruesome and hideous images as well as a constant repetitive barrage of negative no hope statistics all of which conclude with absolute pessimism (true to life or otherwise), and guess what happens to the no hiding place recipients?

Mental Health! An essay! And a bit of history to contemplate.

The most talked about subject this side of Brexit and Covid-19 and the re-decoration of Boris's flat, but why, all of a sudden, has it become such a never-ending high profile topic? As an opener, try defining who exactly is a person with 'mental health issues'. What are the symptoms? What sort of help do we need to make us well and banish the mental health demon? Who will provide all the presumed treatment? What are their qualifications? Will I always have 'issues', and when will I be better? What is the difference between having mental health issues and feeling down and a little depressed? Where has the condition come from, because it appears all of a sudden, that we have pandemic proportions? Now, I can't answer any of those hastily written questions, but the last question i.e. where all of a sudden has the condition materialised from, is for me the most intriguing, because it seems just a few years ago it either didn't exist, or, if it did, why had I (and countless others) never heard of it, or at least never heard it described as it is now, apparently, or so we're reliably informed every day, there are now 'millions' of us confined within its confusing grasp! It was here by-the-way before Covid-19 arrived.

I pondered at length whether to include anything at all in this book on the subject of '*mental health* and *well-being*', and after some thought, was swayed by the fact that as it is currently such an everyday 'hot topic', decided that because 'anything that affects the mental side of life also affects the physical side', there was a place somewhere here for inclusion. The body and the mind are clearly related and part of the same system, the term occasionally used is they are 'indelibly linked', and they work very closely in tandem together, similar perhaps to a footballing striker who has to rely on his winger to accurately cross the ball which enables a goal to be scored, so as with all partners (in this case the head and the body beneath it), one supplies and complements the other, a two way team that works in unison – split the two and we wouldn't be the same species as we are, nor would strikers score so many goals without the winger. And so here are a few humourless issues to muse over.

I must state, before giving some personal views, and as you'll know by now I'm not really 'professionally' qualified in this particular field (apart from age, experiences and life generally), in other words what I mean is I'm clearly not a qualified Doctor, Scientist, Professor or Psychologist; in fact, I'm no different from anyone else, all I have are views, but views which are derived from life's experiences in both sport and life in general. As with all other material in this book, the following views are all mine and of course as I've said before they don't make me right, or popular for that matter, and may even make me unpopular, but that's life, and that's what happens when you extol a view that many others are bound to disagree with! People with views these days are there to be shot at, they're not shrugged off with an 'oh well' comment as they once were. However, just like a lot of the material in this book, my views, and I've seen much, are derived from my 70 years of existence on Planet Earth, I live in the real world a long way from medical couches and laboratories, social hand-outs, celebrities and 'stars', as such I just listen and watch as it all goes around invariably influencing me one way or another before culminating in a personal view. I have though, a mass of practical involvement in life, all accumulated whilst dealing and working alongside a wide variety of people and clearly it is the latter experience which results in most of my views. As close as I've come to subject certification in any way related to mental health is by being a qualified 'Mental Health First Aider' at work (passed the course, got the certificate), I also have a Diploma in Sports Psychology, and am a qualified Counsellor (I'm clearly clutching at straws with all three – nevertheless!). Involvement with real people though is the greatest learning curve, and if I hadn't lived my life the way I have (as far as sporting issues is concerned) as a one person team, presumably I would be just copying other people's views, theories and practices.

One of the real positives with age is the obvious: you've lived longer than many! In an earlier chapter I talked about 'going back' in time i.e. that was within the chapter I'd labelled *'Once Upon a Time'* which seemed like a logical place to go to before moving in the opposite direction and going forward in time and progressing right up to the present, in so doing, I hoped, giving consideration to both the good and the not so good of the past, having been there myself, regardless, when discussing the *mental health* issue which is currently 'so very prevalent *everywhere'*, so let's go back in time again just as a starter, for comparing situations, in any field, allows for a boat load of deliberation.

For people of my generation, that's those of us born in the years just after the Second World War, and more so perhaps those hardened people who preceded me and came before WWII, as well as some with earlier footholds in the years of the 1920s and 1930s and wow how life has changed so considerably since those times. You can only but guess how it must have been for so many young men in the years between 1914 and 1918 all those years ago, to be taken, without fuss or demonstrations, from their chosen or more likely necessary employment and drafted straight into enforced conscription with the armed forces for the sole purpose of fighting for their country in two horrendous World Wars. Living in those times and out of desperation, there were the repercussions of work-related national strikes and with few unions (as yet without much clout) to back up and support the workers. Poverty has 'always' existed (although the meaning of 'poverty' just like the term 'bullying' is varied and open now to wide degrees of interpretation) and was the norm in Victorian times and the early decades of the nineteenth and twentieth centuries. Hard times created by low and unnegotiable wages, with little in the way of social welfare support, as exists in today's society. Thinking back momentarily, I went to school with some kids who had 11 brothers and sisters and some who had to borrow football boots to represent the school; it seems likely, all things considered, in today's ever vigilant social life, that borrowing boots would be highly frowned upon, but the same casual act was never given a second thought in the 1950s. If boots weren't available, then canvas sandshoes would be used to slide all over the field while chasing the elusive ball. Additionally and going back to the 1920/30s and even 1940s, there was little in the way of a meaningful benefit system. No-one (apart from the gentry) had even heard of holidays abroad, but now we are obsessed with them, and tied housing often went hand-in-hand with the job – if you died or lost your job you were literally out on the streets with your family without a roof over your heads. If you had a house, it was always rented or tied in with the job. General living facilities were by modern day standards shocking, with outside privies (emptied by a bloke with a long shovel and a horse and cart), and newspapers were used for toilet roll. Outside in the lane there was the customary communal cold water stand-pipe used by an entire street, and back yards all had tin baths hanging from a nail on the wall because internal bathrooms didn't exist, so bathing was done next to an old black oven in the kitchen. There was no National Health Service until 5th July 1948, (just before I was born – was I lucky or what?) and so with little money to pay for any potential treatment, you either did without or you suffered. Infant death rates were high; most births were carried out in the front room of the house assisted by well-meaning but unqualified neighbours. If you're lucky and live in the North East and want to explore more, visit Beamish Museum in County Durham and you'll get a better grasp of the general living standards of the not too distant past. *As the saying goes, and by comparison, most of us today 'don't know we're born'!* Following the horrendous First World War, where 'millions' were massacred and countless others were terribly mutilated beyond recognition all in the defence of their country folk's freedom, those who survived the quagmire of warfare in those trenches returned home afterwards with most just carrying on life from where they left off, back down the pits (coal mines), or back into heavy industry on key-sides, or working the land etc.* and in those desperate times it seems people had never heard of *mental health issues.* How far have we come? Well, *by contrast there was a small article in today's paper, (and this sort of thing isn't unusual) stating that the BBC is offering counselling to staff 'upset' at the death of Prince Philip!* Unbelievable! Presumably if they weren't offered that costly 'support' they'd just go home and cry, before having a few days off on the sick to recover! On television last week there was a lady who was raising issues about how many women now required mental health support having gone through the 'horrors' of childbirth, I've attended a couple and god knows it isn't easy (an understatement) but why now?

*We have (my family) an ancient small leather pouch, containing two bullets which were removed from my paternal grandad's body during fighting in the trenches of the First World War. Two bullets, a piece of old cloth (possibly from his mother), and a tiny pencil, his belongings! He was the most laid-back, decent, unassuming man you'd ever meet, and would, on the odd occasion the subject was raised, with a nod and a half-smile say, 'I was one of the lucky ones, Michael!' because he came back. He crawled, while seeking help and wounded by all accounts, through waist high mud, in no-man's land, with the two rounds bedded deep inside him. After the hasty field medical 'operation' he was sent home on a train back to England's green and pleasant land, patched up properly in a military hospital, then handed a walking stick to help him get around (we still have it, the cane, from 1916), and then they sent him back to the trenches.

When the war was over, he didn't get 'counselling', or 'mental health' treatment – you know what he did, just like thousands of others, well; he just went back to work to earn an honest living! Then straight after the First World War was over, along came a pandemic occasionally referred to as the Spanish Flu Pandemic and an estimated 50,000,000 people died. Then twenty short years after that there was another World War, and off they all went again!! And here we are in 2021, and we're desperately worried because we may not get a holiday abroad this year, worse again the boozer is still shut, and these issues are apparently contributing to more serious mental health problems, because people 'deserve' a holiday, and a pint or three!

So, here we are in the twenty first century, no pits (coal mines), little in the way of heavy back-breaking industry, being forced to import foreign workers in to pick fruit and veg because we won't do it. That's regardless of all the 'essential' considerable amounts of available mod cons all designed to make life as easy and as comfortable as possible for us, and there is a continuous staggering rise in people with 'mental health' issues. We're 'continually' reminded of this by a repetitive and reoccurring everyday narrative on mental health which accompanies a never-ending analysis surrounding what appears to be of epidemic proportions with millions of people suffering with *mental health* issues which for many of us are an incomprehensible and confusing enigma, on the basis of 'where has it all come from?'. Children as young as nine years of age are giving interviews on television about their, and I quote, 'anxiety attacks'! Now, and I'll say it again, until relatively recent times, I had never heard of people with 'mental health issues', oh, I knew, and indeed know some people had/have bad days and some suffer from occasional bouts of depression, but, over the past few years the phenomenal rise of people claiming to have mental health issues is simply staggering. Every day the subject is aired at great length by television, radio, newspapers, magazines, and even some of our Royalty are not exempt from this modern day 'contagious plague' – as a consequence some 'suffering' yet 'well-heeled' individuals out of desperation find the need to move from a £2,000,000 (plus) house in the country (a gift) to an £11,000,000 house in California to 'escape' their mental health torture. Despite all the information on mental health, much of which is extolled by a never-ending list of professionals with rather grand occupational labels, the subject remains a confusing, sad and expensive everyday discussed topic. Every Sunday we get a newspaper with an attached glossy magazine. The front cover always portrays an attractive female (beauty is in the eye of the beholder, of course) celebrity posturing, made-up to the nines, resplendent in eye catching clothing and make-up complemented with the obligatory gleaming white, even teeth, who then precede through another interview to bemoan on several pages how depressed she is, or has been. Apparently, some want to throw themselves in front of buses, others cry themselves to sleep, some are incredibly depressed by all accounts and seek all means of specialist help, and all, so it seems, have or have had mental health issues ('fortunately' they are keen to share with us –aren't we lucky?).All despite their apparent comfortable wealthy life styles, and so it goes on. In today's paper, and conveniently advertised on the front cover, an everyday presenter, whose husband is extremely ill, has still found time to write a 'soul wrenching' book on her fears and desperations, a great read by all accounts and all yours for £20. Wonder where the purchased books end up once read? Even top professional sports people 'catch it' (mental health issues) and shout for help, both in dealing with their depression during their 'athletic' careers, and then needing more assistance when their sporting lives are over to help them adjust back to 'normal' life once the glory years are gone! We never heard of any of that until recently; I'll say it again, it's *contagious*, the more the subject is raised, the more people 'catch it'. The Olympics are just around the corner – will they bring joy, something to cheer us up or perhaps gloom? One of our current top sprinters has appeared in today's press saying that if he wins a medal he intends to 'take-the-knee' and has 'warned' the International Olympic Committee that 'all hell will break loose' if they dare to sanction anyone who joins the Black Lives Matter protest, and it all 'could go sour very quickly' – and here's me looking forward to 'sport'. Wonder what he's going to do when he can't run fast anymore? How infuriatingly sad, that such a wonderful occasion is to be used for another political statement! The 'everyday' news programmes have worried presenters interviewing depressed people as they saunter slowly along a beautiful beach or in a leafy park, as they're caught by the camera looking 'pretty glum' as they gaze forlornly over the blue sea's horizon; the good news is it must keep musicians in work because the sad people are seemingly always accompanied by the 'oh so sad piano player' tinkering with a musical lament in the background beside the gulls and blackbirds, bet that poor sod (the musician) needs help too, he's bound to catch it if only by association! Once the show case is concluded, there's the customary extended documentary looking at 'the rise in loneliness, depression and 'general' mental health' issues! Tell you what, I write much more on this theme, and I'll be adding to the millions.

Nearly finished. The youth of today though are my biggest concern, simply because they are the future, and if they are so flaming miserable, insecure, and lonely now, well, god help them later when they are cut loose into the real world away from the safe sanctuary of the classroom. Kids are potentially the most robust people on the planet, probably because so early in their lives they have no past to tarnish their young lives. When I was growing up nothing bothered us for long; part of that was due to discipline, and not having options, consequently simply doing what we were told. We knew no different, which was presumably good news for our future employers. Now I truly love children, they invariably make me smile, but what bothers me a little, and I say a little, because there is nothing I can do about it, is mollycoddling children just 'too much', that'll go down like a lead balloon, ouch! I mean the life they inherit after growing up is not easy. Most kids have recently returned to school after the lock-down; however, they don't just 'turn up', and continue where they 'left off', they are carefully escorted by worried parents, and once in the school grounds, the kids are clapped (applauded) into the school yard before getting a reassuring cuddle from the staff, or having a shoulder tenderly rubbed by a concerned supervisory hand, and only then do they begin their lessons (what must the kids be thinking?). By contrast, have a look at the migration camps around the Middle East and elsewhere, thousands living in tattered make-shift tents, up to their knees in mud with little in the way of basic sanitation, if you are my age the whole situation is mind boggling. The words 'mental health' are a relatively modern day term, I use the 'modern day' term, and I've said it before, because it wasn't around when I was at school, and even for most of my years as an adult and right up to fairly recent times, if we were sad we were told to 'cheer up and get over it' – end of; now there'd be major concerns that the unsmiling child is suffering from serious health issues. During my years in the

Royal Marines, I truly can't remember the subject even being raised, let alone debated and we were 'trained' to be 'first in and last out' while operating in the killing fields of the world!

My view, and bear with me I'll be coming to a sharp conclusion soon, is that, if we wake up to a 'never-ending' daily onslaught of references revolving around mental health issues (see the link to Buddy Guy mentioned above), and we are continually reminded of the same every five minutes throughout the 24-hour day, while at the same time bombarded with mysterious, difficult to define symptoms, which are cascaded by people with faces all screwed up in apparent misery, then because of its habitual never-ending mantra it all becomes by association **contagious,** and because we all mingle, well sooner or later we're just bound to 'catch it', just like we would if we were holed-up in an airless room with the virus.

The every-day news has no 'good' news, I mean in a 30-minute programme, there's none, and everything is 'bad' news. Today, 7/4/21, a prominent news headline on mainstream television refers to an epidemic of 'loneliness' sweeping the country, particularly among the old and the young; are the figures correct? And where do all the eye-catching numbers come from? Then there's the never-ending and unescapable television adverts which come up every five minutes between an overwhelming abundance of morbid hell-fire documentaries and extremely violent plays and films, some of the charity adverts are absolutely shocking and they aren't on 'after' the one-time important 9 o'clock watershed. Soaps haven't escaped; they are a never-ending day to day life of so called 'ordinary' people whose lives are little other than total misery, clearly any type of humour is now banned, presumably because it could 'offend'. Talking of humour, there's a recent programme about to arrive which asks the question *'what is funny?'* – Ha! Tell you what, get the answer wrong and you could end up in jail while being labelled some sort of 'ist. Here's the best advice? Only laugh when the rest of them laugh – that's the way to do it, Micky son, that'll keep you out of the slammer, eh? Or at least you'll go there with some more like-minded people. Now I am an animal and bird loving softy, animal cruelty and abuse as graphically described in endless charity adverts really affect me big time and it doesn't matter how many times 'I have to see them', I always see them with the same amount of horror as I see or hear about child abuse. These advertisements are on relentlessly and unless you are sitting with the remote, there is nowhere to escape them; even when you've joined the charities and paid your monthly fees, you are still repeatedly subjected to the same graphic horrors several times a day, isn't that a type of indoctrination? I must have seen some of them hundreds of times. If you somehow miss the animal and human abuse ones, up will pop your favourite household celebrity desperate to earn yet another buck by any means available as they cascade the never-ending costs of Funerals whilst asking you if you've got yours ready and paid for because it's coming – give me a break! Other celebs and once proud sports stars sit morosely with their trousers rolled up around their knees enjoying a vibrator work-out and would seemingly 'love to go for a walk' – but because of some form of 'age related' disability they're not able, until they use some miracle cream or purchase a wonderful vibrating machine specifically designed to caress their pins. You know what, when I was growing up you got the news at 6pm and again around 9pm; contrast that with every minute of the day 24/7 twelve months of the year. Whatever happened to the sprightly tuneful jingles that accompanied the smiling laddie with *"don't forget the fruit gums, mum!"* and the dentists' receptionist with the perfect 'false teeth' crooning *'you'll wonder where the yellow went when you brush your teeth with Pepsodent!' Oh to hear again the jaunty 'the Esso sign means happy motoring, the Esso sign means happy motoring' etc or the grown-up Scottish and Newcastle beer advert which had the fat guy jovially singing 'wherever you go you're sure to find a Blue Star' ha ha I'm feeling better already!!* Even now 60-plus years later, they make me smile at the innocence and newness of it all! You want to take the knee? Go ahead, but presumably we can still take the knee while smiling, instead of looking like a bunch of 'poorly paid gladiators' waiting for the Lions, now those poor buggers (gladiators and Christians alike) would have good reason for catching the mental health bug!

I see and hear the youth of today being interviewed on television, words are put into their mouths by the interviewer by simply asking the leading question *"how has your 'mental health' been during the pandemic while you've been 'off school' and 'absent from your friends' and wider family? It must have been so hard for you?"* after the latter, a reply is unlikely to render a jovial *"oh wonderful, an extra holiday whoopee, it's been really good, my keepy-ups have improved immeasurably and I've learned to read and peel tetties with me gran, thanks very much for asking".* The kids have all the modern day terminology that goes with the terrain; they are deeply ingrained, because there's no escape, as well as 'anxiety attacks' apparently many get 'panic attacks', who told them about those modern day scourges affecting the young. Torture of military personnel when captured is similar, a 'bombardment' of repetitive loud music and a Lord Haw-Haw (William Joyce) giving his endless prophesies of doom which is purposely designed to torture, to crack the detainee resulting in giving the foe all the info they require. The difference is that during the war years Mr Haw-Haw was cheerfully laughed at and ridiculed probably while sitting freezing on an outside 'netty', a good entertaining comedy, not to be missed. Talking of comedies, it's well known that laughing is a real tonic, and a good comedy was/is worth its weight in gold, not now though; the good comedies of my youth and beyond are banned because 'someone' somewhere finds them 'offensive'! What about the millions who don't find them in the least bit offensive? Surely the minority can turn the channel over, if they can find where they've hidden the remote. Oh what a sad chapter this has been, I'm sorry, and by the way I love kids, Victor Meldrew has nothing on me, eh? Hang-on, just seen another mind boggling stat which has just weaved its way over the bottom part of the television, 50,000 reported sexual assaults in our universities! Can't think of anything to add!!!

The problem is, I suppose, can we ever get back to what was once normal, where taking the rough with the smooth was an everyday 'chore', and regardless we coped because there was no other option. 'I'm having a bad day; I'm feeling a bit down' and 'I've a terrible headache' were part of 'normal' life. The throw away, 'Oh roll on Friday' was generally met with a supporting nod and subdued smile, today the latter universal throw-away 'quip' would be identified as a 'warning sign' by the much respected (and feared) in-house Mental Health First Aider (bet you wouldn't come to me eh?) who will accompany you to the psychologist's bench at the sick bay, where Elastoplasts and bandages have been replaced with drawers full of mental health books and walls full of scary posters forbidding us the urge to smile and make Jokes.

My advice?

We are all but specks of sand in the desert, as such soon to move on to wherever the wind takes us. In just a hundred years from now, 99.9 percent of the current population will be gone, billions of us will have left, now that kind of puts it all into a bit of perspective, don't you think? Try not to see yourself as too important – one thing is for sure – many of us are lucky to be here, if only for a short while! Make the most of it, and don't burden others with either repetitive, never-ending statistics or morbidity in general.

Whilst I feel somewhat uneasy writing the latter 'views', I get a small amount of comfort from the thought that books of this nature can perhaps be viewed as a 'historical document' if only because they come from a specific time, as such they may act as an up-to-date view of life in 2021 United Kingdom, whilst allowing a comparison of both the past and the future! Finally, many of us are trying desperately to hang onto the principle of a society which still values 'freedom of speech' and the right to hold a view even if it's fundamentally different from the views and opinions of others, so as such try to refrain from chucking clods of earth my way – wasted anyhow, because currently I'm still fit enough to dodge them! God bless you all, I really like you!

AND NOW FOR SOMETHING A BIT DIFFERENT AND MORE IN LINE WITH THE INTENDED SUBJECT MATERIAL.

Test your health and fitness general knowledge!

Q1: Heart disease still accounts for a third of all deaths in the UK, name four common causes of heart disease?

A1: In no specific order: Obesity, poor diet, stress, lack of exercise, high blood pressure, smoking, excessive drinking. Some of the above don't cause heart disease by themselves, rather they can 'contribute' to the condition.

Q2: Briefly outline the importance of the heart and its function.

A2: The heart is a muscular pump responsible for life itself! Quality of life is governed to a degree, by its working efficiency. Its function is to pump blood and circulate blood around the body. Within the blood are oxygen and nutrients essential for life itself.

Q3: What are carbohydrates? Briefly describe their nutritional value.

A3: Carbohydrates are energy-giving foods and drinks. There are two types of carbohydrates:

1. Complex

   Very good for us, high in energy, low in fat, high in vitamins, high in minerals and high in fibre. Complex carbohydrates include: Wholemeal products such as pasta, rice, cereals (porridge etc.) fruit, vegetables, etc.

2. Simple

> Still high in energy, but of a quick burning type, they are also low in nutritional value, high in refined white sugar, few if any vitamins and minerals, high in calories, simple carbohydrates include confectionery bars, sweets, cakes, biscuits, fizzy drinks etc.

Q4: Dairy produce is made up of what nutritional source?

A4: **Fat! Not all bad though. There are also a variety of vitamins and minerals (including calcium). Remember fat is partly responsible for 'furring up' of blood vessels, ultimately resulting in blockages of the blood vessels, potentially leading to Myocardial Infarction (heart attacks).**

Q5: Which of the following meats has less fat? Beef, Chicken or Lamb.

A5: **Chicken has less fat, but you should remove the skin. It pays to remember that even lean cuts of meat can have a high proportion of fat which may not be visible. Beware of products such as Hamburgers, Sausages, Bacon, and kebabs. Meat products can also be difficult to digest – they can 'hang around' for lengthy periods.**

Q6: Which of the following cheeses has less fat? Edam, cottage or cheddar.

A6: **Cottage cheese followed by Edam.**

Q7: Name 3 foods high in Vitamin C.

A7: **Fruit and vegetables, including citrus fruits – oranges/grapefruit/lemon, strawberries, raspberries, potatoes and a variety of vegetables.**

Q8: Vitamin C is water soluble – true or false?

A8: TRUE. Vitamin C is water soluble meaning it dissolves in liquid and is therefore secreted by the body with water (urine/sweat); as a result the vitamin can't be stored, therefore daily amounts are required to keep levels up and maintain good health. Depending on your diet, a Vitamin C supplement can be taken.

Q9: Identify three foods high in fibre.

A9: Complex Carbohydrates such as wholemeal bread, fruit, vegetables, wholemeal cereals, lentils, beans etc. There is a very obvious and common theme here – complex carbs! Much of the fibre is in the skin so keep it on with apples, pears, even 'baked' potatoes harbour more Vitamin C and fibre.

Q10: Why is fibre important in your diet?

A10: Fibrous foods (anything with skin on the outside) are good for your internal digestive system. They also add bulk to your food, which tends to make you feel 'full', limiting excess. Fibrous food also goes through the digestive system quicker.

IT'S A PITY, IN MY OPINION, THAT CARBOHYDRATES OFTEN HAVE SO MUCH BAD PRESS. THEY ARE NUTRIONALLY VERY SOUND, PROVIDE A LOT OF VITAMINS AND MINERALS AND ARE HIGH IN ENERGY. PLUS, THEY ARE GENERALLY CHEAP TO BUY; ADDITIONALLY, MANY OF THE PRODUCTS ARE EASY TO GROW. BUT BE WARY OF 'SIMPLE' CARBS, THEY AREN'T SO GOOD, PITY THEY OFTEN TASTE SO NICE! OH WELL, A LITTLE OF WHAT YOU FANCY EH?

Q11: Name three of the most health-promoting breakfast cereals?

A11: Porridge, shredded wheat, Weetabix, muesli with no added sugar are some of the better ones, nutritionally sound and low in refined white sugar and salt – if you want to sweeten your bowl up a bit try adding bananas, strawberries, raspberries, blueberries, grapes or dried fruit.

Q12: Identify an exercise you consider to be the optimum in physical training; make an 'objective' choice.

A12: A highly debateable question as there are so many forms of exercise to choose from. Rowing is amongst the best for an all-round workout, jogging/running, swimming, cycling are also very good but for different reasons; with some of the latter you should consider additional upper-body exercises to complement them. DON'T FORGET WALKING – WE TALKED QUITE A BIT ON THAT EARLIER, BUT TRY NOT TO SAUNTER TOO MUCH OTHERWISE YOUR CARDIO WILL REMAIN PRETTY MUCH DORMANT. REMEMBER, AEROBIC EXERCISE IS GOOD FOR YOUR ENGINE BUT OPERATING TOO SLOW WILL LIMIT THE BENEFIT.

Q13: Give reasons for your choice in question 12.

A13: An optimum exercise should be one that is considered for its all-round qualities, i.e. cross training covers a multitude of activities, as does the sport of triathlon. Aerobic (heart, lungs, circulation), Strength (to improve muscular efficiency), Flexibility (improve or maintain your range of movement). Risk of injury potential should also be a consideration, and finally last but not least 'Longevity' should also be one of your main aims, meaning 'how long' are you prepared to keep your choice in your life, the harder or more difficult you find something, the more the likelihood of you discontinuing. All things considered, my own preference would be for rowing (however, there is a boredom issue, particularly for static room type rowing) due to its all-round conditioning effect, although I'm not a rower myself (I did say objective!). It is worth noting that non-weight bearing activities create a lesser injury risk on the basis that there are no impact elements, i.e. body to surface and stress. But with non-impact activities there are little in the way of bone strengthening – it sounds contradictory; however, bones in your skeletal frame need impact of sorts to maintain their strength, impact is necessary for healthy bones.

A combination of exercises is best, providing they suit the individual, i.e. someone who is shorter in height perhaps 5'2" and weighs 18 stone would be ill advised to choose running! So careful consideration is essential when choosing an exercise programme. My advice is base your choice on 'longevity'; short term pain and discomfort does not encourage continuation.

Q14: What does the term 'Aerobic' mean?

AQ14: The term 'aerobic' simply means an exercise whereby the body's demand for oxygen is met, and you aren't unduly out of breath. So it is basically 'steady state' exercise, keeping breathing and heart rates steady throughout the exercise. Typically jogging/running, swimming, cycling, rowing, aerobics classes, stepping, dancing which increases heart rate to ensure you are getting the desired training effect. Aerobic exercise is great for the cardio-vascular system.

Q15: A low resting pulse would normally indicate what?

AQ15: A low resting pulse rate normally indicates an efficient cardio-vascular system, i.e. the heart is performing well with little in the way of effort. Although it does vary, age also plays a role, a normal resting heart rate for an adult with no known ailments, would be around 70-80 beats per minute. Endurance sportspeople regularly have pulse rates in the high 30s or low to mid 40s (even at 70 years of age my resting HR is between 45-48 bpm) which would signify their hearts pumping action satisfies their body's demand for energy (through the transference of oxygen carrying blood) for a reduced amount of work because every beat is powerful enough to satisfy the body's demand.

Taking your pulse rate regularly once you've started an exercise programme is an ideal way of monitoring your physical progress, as your heart becomes stronger through regular exercise, its pumping action slows, indicating it is doing more but for less effort.

Q16: Abdominal exercise will enable me to lose weight around my stomach – true or false?

A16: False! This is a common misconception. The body burns fat as an energy source 'centrally' or as a whole. You cannot target individual areas to reduce body fat by specifically working an individual section. If we work aerobically while reducing our food and drink intake, the law of averages says we must sooner or later begin to shred weight. However, as a result of the weight loss, folds of skin may materialise. As a means of improving our appearance (if indeed that's important to you) toning up the muscles underneath the folds is advised i.e. abdominal exercises for the stomach or bicep curls and triceps extensions for the arms should give better definition, therefore a leaner, fitter appearance with some muscular definition should be the end result. In summary, burn body fat whilst exercising aerobically while also firming up the limbs and stomach with an array of resistance exercises is a sound formula, but it has to be said, it won't happen overnight, it takes time and consistent effort.

Q17: For the average person (if there is such a thing) what is the recommended amount of sleep per 24 hours?

A17: At the time of writing this one's a hot potato. The fact is that we all vary so much – for some four hours appears to work fine, for others 10 hours appears normal, but on average the consensus is that around 7 to 8 hours is the norm and should do the job. Any less than what is 'normal for the individual' may lead to irritability, lower working capacity mentally as well as physically. It's important to state that most physical improvement deriving from exercise takes place while the body is resting, not when it's active, the harder or more you exercise the more recovery needed, until your body adjusts to the stress applied. As I write we are being consistently told that a lack of sleep may lead to an increased possibility of dementia. Now the latter information is not likely to lead to a better night's sleep, is it? In my world as I look for answers, I have often used children as an interesting guide, that's because they do what comes naturally, that's before society steps in to create a 'what is acceptable culture'. Grown-ups are different, we aren't as instinctively bright. Kids seem to get the formula right, they sleep when they're tired, comfortable and stress free, when they are tense, excited, agitated or even unhappy they struggle. Me? I've been a poor sleeper all my life, despite my extreme seventy years of daily exercise, I've come to terms with it, as it seems there is little I can do to promote sleep, apart from take some pills – and I'LL NOT DO THAT.

Q18: Your last meal before exercise should be (a) 45 minutes, (b) 2 hours, (c) 3hrs 30mins?

A18: At least two hours, although light snacks should not interfere too much. Drinking regular small amounts of water is beneficial to remain hydrated and should not interfere with your exercise.

Q19: Regarding question 18, briefly identify why.

A19: The obvious purpose of food and drink is to provide energy, growth, insulation, repair etc. However, it takes a period of time from ingestion to result in these functions. During the early part of digestion the food lies passively in the stomach, where it resides as a dead weight of no particular value. Also, digestion requires blood, so a good proportion of blood is directed to the gut from other areas, e.g. leg and arm muscles. So just at that crucial moment when we start to exercise and therefore need all the energy we can get, we are heavily restricted because of our recent meal. It also pays to remember that fats and proteins take longer to digest than a meal high in carbohydrates. Meats and dairy play little part in initial energy production.

Q20: A sugary drink prior to exercise will enhance my physical performance. True or False?

A20: False. Within the bloodstream, circulating around the body, we have what can be described as 'sensory hormones' which detect physiological changes in the body such as temperature or sugar levels. Depending on the detection, corrective action is automatically taken to maintain a correct balance. Shivering or sweating are two typical reactions.

When we have a sudden influx of sugar into the bloodstream, via a sugary drink or confectionery, this is quickly identified and a process of reducing the sugar levels is put into operation. However, because of the high level of sugar there can be an over-reaction which may result in too much sugar being removed from the bloodstream into the liver, so at the commencement of exercise, our initial energy source is non-existent. As a result, when we start to exercise we are quickly short of fuel, which is perhaps not what you'd expect having purposefully taken an 'energy' drink! Following several minutes of exercise, depending on the duration of the activity, it can be beneficial to 'top up' with a regular intake of carbohydrate. The Great North Run is a good example of when energy top-ups are beneficial.

Q21: The following body parts are frequently injured during physical training – where would you find them? (A) Achilles Tendon, (B) Patella, (C) Clavicle, (D) Lumbar vertebrae.

A21: Achilles tendon – Ankle to Calf; Patella – Knee; Clavicle – Shoulder; Lumbar vertebrae – Back.

Q22: What is a clear sign of dehydration?

A22: A good indication of low water levels is the colour of your urine; ideally a clear transparent colour is best, as opposed to a rusty colour. Water is one of the most health-promoting elements available. Most people

drink far too little resulting in a mild form of dehydration. In men, up to 65% of the body is made up of water; in women, up to 55%. It's therefore obvious that a water deficiency will result in below-par efficiency.

Q23: What does the term 'passive smoking' mean?

A23: All workplaces now have a no smoking policy in certain defined areas. The policy is designed to protect non-smokers from the unpleasant and dangerous effects of inhaling smoke projected from either the cigarette held in the hand or the smoke exhaled from the mouth of the smoker. Passive smoking could be described as involuntary participation in a very harmful addiction.

Q24: What is the considered weekly intake of alcohol?

A24: This area has been subject to some debate for years. However, guidelines issued by the Health Education Authority are that males and females should keep alcohol intake down to 14 units per week which equates to seven pints of beer or 14 single measures of spirits or wine.

Q25: Gluteus Maximus was a Roman Emperor. True or False?

Q25: Emperors?!!! Gluteus Maximus is your buttocks!

ASK QUESTIONS!

TO: Daniel, and Joe Dixon, the world is your oyster – don't ever end up wondering! Good luck!

Over the past few years, I've been assisting a very promising young triathlete called Daniel Dixon to attain his athletic potential. From the onset of our relationship I have encouraged him to be always inquisitive, in other words don't just accept advice, analyse it, and then if you don't understand why you are doing a form of training at a particular time, ask, don't just accept it all without sound reasoning. The question should always be – 'what will I gain by that?' If I struggle for an answer, you have every right to be suspicious.

I would recommend the same sentiments for everybody who seeks advice from 'professionals'. Guff advice has always existed and there can be little doubt that a lot of time is wasted due to well-intentioned but misdirected or ill-informed advice. I do believe that people who query or question are in most cases not obstructive as may be perceived, but probably have a higher degree of intellect or personal interest. Certainly, none of us should buy a product without analysing its potential!

CONCLUSION – Almost!

I've tried very hard not to turn this book into a 'replica' of so many others; however, there are some things which regardless of how you dress them up, well they are simply fact. I mean 'interval training' is interval training, and 'Weetabix is a complex carbohydrate', and 'hamstrings run down the back of your legs' and you can't change any of those, because they are fact, like 5 plus 5 equals 10. However, using my own life and personal experiences, which are really quite vast, I hope has allowed me a differing take on many things. Isn't the chapter on mental health a grind? I apologise again! But that's the way I see it, as a nation we've gone soft, you know colds aren't just spread by a virus, they are shared in society by word of mouth 'I have one and you're bound to catch it', and so you do! I believe the growth in mental health issues is similar, we are bombarded endlessly with the subject 24/7 and so people get miserable and become part of the stats. In contrast to my athletic life, so many other authors have little real 'practical' experience although at a glance they appear well enough qualified, either because of the way they look or perhaps by a few written qualifications and the labels that are attached to them, and I have little doubt that some people progress because they have the right 'connections', *but you don't learn to fly a Jet by sitting comfortably in a hangar while analysing aviation rules and regulations for a later test!* What is interesting, I hope, is 'being successful' in my own small way, while at the same time having the nerve to continually *'buck the trends'* while treading lesser known tracks and pathways to get to my perceived destination! Nobody ever cared, very few asked or enquired, but that was all part of my incentive; those who did ask didn't understand anyhow!

My life has always been a contradiction, and with me, what people see has always been clouded by my competitive 'athletic life' and the thousands of competitions (and outstanding results) I've endlessly done for my entire life.

Each one of those countless competitions were for me, a little like a 'job interview' a chance to impress, except that there was no bullshit in either my athletic training or my competitions, they were both so fundamentally honest as I vigorously chased sporting successes, because on conclusion of each event, win or lose, there was ultimately nowhere to hide, the end results were simply an honest statement labelled *look what I've done – didn't I do good*! I am not alone in the last expression, and many are similar to me. In contrast, and unlike a 'job interview', there was no requirement for meaningless pieces of run-of-the-mill written attainment certification primarily designed so others could put a tick in an appropriate box. Training and competitions didn't require any false enforced smiles and pleasantries, accompanied by cosy handshakes, nor perfected and practised words or audible specialist bull-shitting terminology; neither were presentable best suits with matching shiny ties necessary, or deceitful clever nods of agreement designed to fit the placement. For me, all my athletic attainments were incredibly sincere, I didn't know how to cheat and I view them all as a kind of 'character assessment'; the shiny suits required at the interview with hints of aftershave were replaced with sweat-soaked flimsy cotton vests and skin deep, 'no hiding place', honest, difficult to hide emotions. When the gun sounds the start of the race – you are alone; that's what I like about individual sports.

In life, almost *everything is a contradiction of something* – e.g. 'don't eat eggs but increase your protein', or – 'calcium is vital for bone strength and maintenance – but don't eat dairy produce because it's high in fat', 'jogging is great for your cardio but it'll hammer your pins!'etc. *Another 'contradiction' which is 'almost' funny is people's absolute 'obsession' with staying alive at all costs, yet the very same people are too lethargic to take even the lowest levels of health promoting nutrition and then complement the food and drink with even minimal amounts of easy to do exercise – if only to 'maintain 'that magical gift of health', that personal gift that enables a full and interesting life.* People will wear masks to protect themselves from the virus, yet at the same time continue to poison themselves while smoking bucket loads of carbon monoxide and drinking to excess. People will willingly swallow a mountain of tablets to stay alive, yet at the same time continue to ingest dubious food and drink which is contributing big style to their demise. People have been informed that heart disease for most people is preventable and the condition is due to poor health choices, yet the same people, who fear death like a penalty in the Gallowgate End in extra time, refuse to take the 'simplest' of initiatives to improve their chances. Still talking contradictions, people are encouraged to exercise, yet refuse to leave the sofa and go outside in case the virus chases them down, 'trips them from behind' and gives them a sopping wet kiss, then when the pandemic 'is all over' and we all come out the other end and return to normality, the same people who have been so guarded against the virus can now barely walk, because they've hidden under the bed with a mask on for a full year! Apparently, during the pandemic, there has been a noticeable increase in people buying dogs, I wonder how many of those apparent dog lovers will refuse to walk them once the newness has declined and the rain falls – whatever were you thinking buying a Springer when you have a phobia of anything relating to exercise? In all my writings I do attempt to be at least 'rational' and see the world not just as I view it but also to see it all through the eyes of other equals. Although you wouldn't know it, *I do find writing with a critical pen incredibly difficult,* because by nature I'm really not a nasty person, I like to think I'll help anybody. Yet the one thing which is so obvious is many people's inclination to ignore anything and everything that causes them the slightest bit of trouble. At the end of the day, the word that sums up so many of us is *laziness,* an 'I can't be bothered' attitude, which becomes immediately contradictable when their telephone call hurriedly summons help and an ambulance pulls up at the door and the wheels finally take away most of the casualty's previously possessed 'can do options' to be rapidly replaced by 'can't do options'. And when the ambulance brings the person back there's little left, because they've willingly given away the greatest gift of all, which is their irreplaceable good health, and it's never to return.

I wrote the following chapter 21 years ago; nothing, it seems, has changed, except the forsaken freedom of speech we've readily given up, to be replaced by a boat load of boring, incomprehensible political correctness. As I write and finalise this book, and it's just another bewildering day, a Headmistress has forbidden the term 'Good morning boys and girls' to be used in her school! So, where does that leave the Blaydon Races, Miss? Which for the past 100 years plus, had the same 'inappropriate' words 'all the lads and lasses there and all their smiling faces, gannin alang the Scotswood Road' …etc. Go tell it to the Leazes End, Miss!

As so many of my country folk have, by choice, become physically redundant, I often recall another society I observed many years ago and in contrast it went like this. As a rookie Royal Marine back in the early 1970s, I can recall running (with a submachine gun in my hands) between shop doorways while taking part in company exercises in Hong Kong. At about five o'clock in the morning, just as the sun was coming up, I remember being slightly puzzled and a little bemused by the sight of what appeared to be literally hundreds of elderly Chinese people emerging from every 'nook and cranny' in all manners of casual dress as they headed towards communal exercise parks. The intention? To take part in a daily exercise routine, 'before' they commenced a 12 or 16-hour working day. Some had cheap, well-worn flip flops on; others had no footwear at all; and most had a vest and a matching, baggy, ill-fitting pair of shorts or spacious flannel pants. As only marines would, we sniggered and smirked, under the accepted collective opinion that they were all 'dirty stop outs' still half canned from the previous night's merriment.

Anyhow, the scenario must have had an impact on me because I've lived the scene many times since, sometimes with amusement regarding our marine brand of humour (it was ignorance), but also because of an occasional interest in the fundamental beliefs of the working Chinese. On reflection, their philosophies were probably something like, *keep fit today and tomorrow I'll still be able and capable.* I believe I'm right in saying their society at the time had no place for 'hangers on'. If you didn't work, then you didn't eat or provide either, so the incentive to remain fit and 'useful' must have been massive, driven by 'discipline' (a word I've mentioned several times before in this book) based on the harsh reality of living without a great deal of support.

Our own society and current culture would appear to be in total contrast and goes something like 'neglect myself today (because I'm too apathetic or lethargic to do otherwise) and the NHS will take responsibility tomorrow'! The current abundance and never-ending media driven debates, and chat shows and question-time type programmes continually debate the inadequacies of the NHS – no money, no equipment, no staff, not enough beds etc. Because they're in the audience, there's not a word about the 'clientele who inhabit the wards and take up the beds', nor is there ever mention of taking at least some personal responsibility, and many (by no means all) of the latter are where they are through personal neglect and therefore choice. I'm not dressing anyone down, just telling it the way it is – the truth!

Now I would not wish to appear callous because I'm not, but I can tell you there are more 'volunteers' than 'victims' in hospital beds. I'm not prone to making exaggerated statements; however, **most** of our nation are prepared to ignore the health advice and repetitive warnings regarding the massive growth in obesity. A further sign of the times or so I've heard, is a drive, by 'someone' trying to rid the English language of the word obesity because it's offensive – well, take the word away if you must, but you'll have to replace it with something else ('a little teeny weeny bit chubby' – how's that?) simply because the condition still exists, and like it or not obesity is real and it's here, until we change from being obese to 'a little overweight', and the latter can be done if the will is there.

There's nothing that will remove or eradicate ill health and sickness from society altogether, it is part of life, people will get ill, people will age, and accidents are inevitable; additionally, some people are dealt a harsh hand (an under-statement) as far as health is concerned which has little to do with 'fault' and that's why the NHS is such an absolute and treasured gem and an absolute necessity. However, and in conclusion, so many of us have a choice in how we live our lives, and that personal choice will, and does, affect others. For every person taking up a bed in a hospital, it is one less for someone else. With health and fitness 'you reap what you sow'! Pointing the finger elsewhere, often firmly in the back yard of the National Health Service, is totally absurd.

AND FOR THE EPILOGUE

THE AMUSING AND UNAVOIDABLE SUBJECT OF 'AGEING'!

I'VE LEFT THIS OFT REFERRED TO 'TONGUE IN CHEEK' TOPIC RIGHT TILL LAST, IT'S SOMETHING FITTING TO CONCLUDE THIS 'ONE WAY DISCUSSION' WITH, AND THE SUBJECT OF AGING I THINK SITS WELL AS THE EPILOGUE OF THIS BOOK!

For all of us who travel the unavoidable aging highway, there is an uncertain and totally unpredictable future, for just like driving a car in the fog we can't see what awaits around the next bend, so go easy, keep healthy and remain alert if you want to continue a while longer!

Learning from the future is not possible; until it's been and gone, then all too quickly the future has transcended into the present. We should learn well from the past, that's why I have used a lot of it in this self-acknowledged messy publication. The past has much to offer and should never be seen as boring old rubbish. Few people, it seems, are currently interested in old athletes. A short while ago I finished 15th in a 10km race from hundreds (at 68) and didn't get so much as a handshake; tomorrow I am doing a duathlon (at 70) and have just been informed there's no age group prizes, prizes are only for those young enough to win, not that I need yet another trophy, of course, but others might find one something to really celebrate and cherish! Older people seldom feature in the news in the 21st century and I fully understand that. We live in an era whereby visually handsome, pretty people, as well as those who've 'benefited' greatly from a set of brand new teeth as well as a mountain of cosmetic 'refinement' guaranteed to give them a 'presumed' (and open to debate) gorgeous appearance, which in 2021 out-sells almost anything 'meaningful' or real. In contrast, the 'ordinary' elderly are seldom seen as physically attractive and in today's world old age is often seen as an absolute negative. Today's newspaper has given a glimpse of some soon to be issued postal stamps, the stamps are designed to pay homage to Prince Philip having recently died, but all four stamps are of the prince in his youthful good-looking years, none resemble the wonderful elderly gentleman he naturally became as he aged before he died – why?

In terms of movement, quite naturally as we age we gradually move slower than we ever did before, and unless we fight back a little, well sooner rather than later we will be compelled to stop altogether, expectations of society can further speed up the decline. Still talking of the elderly, with little to look forward to, our lives are often immersed in the past which often leads to us being labelled as 'has-beens' who have little new or exciting to offer a modern world, yet much like a 600 year old withering oak tree, many of the elderly have witnessed much and have endured, adjusted, and manoeuvred within times of colossal change, the latter 'change' acting as both our nemesis and our tutor. As an athlete, some, like me, learned our trade as we went because back in the day when 'amateurism' ruled there wasn't an alternative, as such with our learning we clearly became wiser after we broke the tape. Bob Dylan put it so much more eloquently when he said 'you better start swimming or you'll sink like a stone' is – at least for me, a reminder perhaps not to dwell too long on the negativities that accompany the aging process, rather rebel a little while swimming against the tide of change and continue to exercise with a degree of pride because to do so may result in increasing the possibilities of a self-reliance which is far better than 'rest in peace'!

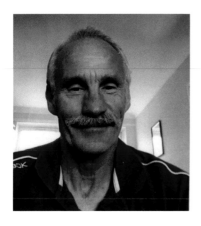

See what Covid did to me! I'm better now though, I've had the jabs and the 'tash' has simply disappeared - and my wife sleeps with me again, isn't it wonderful! - Yippee!

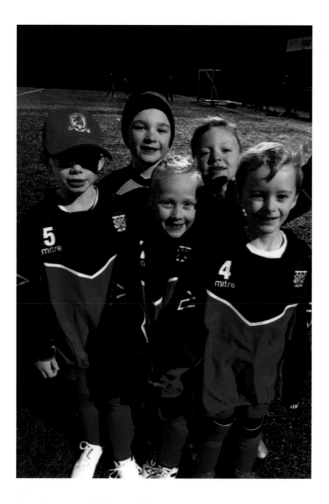

Pope Gregory the Great, whilst walking around a market and coming across several childen, said 'Where are these from', the reply was, 'They are angles' to which he replied, 'These aren't angles' these are angels!' Hah! Read below...

"Grandad, aren't you nearly a hundred?" said a young four year old Dan Harris (in front of several of his worried and concerned little chums!). And young Dan's grandad was heard to reply angrily, "If you ever say that again in public – I'll smack you hard!!" And the kids were heard to whisper, "Has he got a will, the oldies have all got loads of money? BAH, A HUNDRED – IS THAT ALL HE IS!!!"

Aging and getting older is the one thing in our lives whereby we have no personal precedent. I mean we can go backwards and learn from our past, but not forwards and learn from our future – someone will be working on it though, I bet! So, with no precedent to guide us, and depending on your psyche the future is either at best very exciting or at worst horribly daunting. For the elderly, there are few birthday 'yippees' which were once yelled excitedly to greet another exciting new year. As mentioned above, few things it seems are ever greeted positively with increasing age, and any age-based uncertainty is derived around the fact that there is a perceived and unprecedented negative downward 'change' that accompanies getting older. Attempting to quantify 'ageing' is within itself interesting, attempting to quantify aging with a degree of 'positivity' is almost formidable! There are no definitive ageing numbers to put us into a carefully defined category, so as such we go from being seen as a child, then quickly identified as a youth, and once there at what age do you graduate and transfer over and become a recognised adult? Then a short while later we hear a voice whispering in our ever-receptive ear *'look–out middle age is a coming you're 40! – argh – slippers and striped pyjamas beckon, quick – duck, swerve, dive, above all avoid at all costs!'* And following on, the finale is the cringeworthy mantle referred to as 'old age' and at the end of the aging finale – we go to sleep!

For a lot of us our mind is the Governor and our body the supporting Serf who is obliged and conditioned to just follow blindly! Positive in mind, positive in body!

What a piece of work is a man! How noble in reason! How infinite in faculty! In form and moving, how express and admirable! In action how like an angel! In apprehension, how like a god! The beauty of the world! The paragon of animals!

William Shakespeare said that, presumably he wasn't talking about the over 60s – see end of chapter for a personal update!

SO, WHAT'S IT LIKE TO BE 70 YEARS OF AGE AND AN ATHLETE?

As I write, in my 70th year, my athletic *performance* (training and competing) is currently more important than any thoughts about exercise for the purpose of ensuring *longevity, i.e. living for the sake of it, and currently I only want to live a long extended life, on the proviso that I can still laugh 'at everything', whilst being physically able and healthy to do it! I see no joy in being bored rigid, while to ease the blight of loneliness I consider the purchase of another dog to talk lovingly to while whispering sweet nothings into its tentative but scruffy ears, and to kiss and cuddle after one pint too many. Nor do I have any desire to be silently thought of as an unwelcome drain on either family or country.*

The first thing I'd say is that in terms of ageing and sporting issues, it's the body, from the neck downwards, that 'silently' changes, the *mind* which controls us seems like an immovable slave-master, the dictator, and the disciplinarian, which somewhat harshly perhaps, keeps us as competitive as we've always been. The mind doesn't seem to change with age in the same way the body does, nor is it susceptible to bullying as the athletic body is; additionally the mind doesn't seem to be altered or repressed by undeniable logic. As daft as it may sound, providing you train (exercising occasionally for health is different) consistently and you remain injury-free for long periods, I find that *'expectations'* when racing, as well as involvement in other competitive 'games', really don't change that much – what I'm saying is that I still consciously stand on the 'front line' at the start of events, not at the back anticipating an 'also ran' performance. The wonderful act of 'dreaming' has always provided the athlete with motivation – remove the dream and you potentially remove the motivation; regardless, optimism remains a steadfast virtue and an ever dependable friend of the ambitious athlete. Negativity, on the other hand, in all its varying forms is as always the athletes' nemesis and principal foe!

Having said the latter, reality is an irrefutable leveller, and much of reality is the bed-fellow of fact, and for the athlete sporting 'results' are an ever-present and reoccurring factual update, and for the athlete with each passing year after 60 it does seem there are small but noticeable physical changes, For the sporting practitioner, however, there is no doubt that some types of sports are invariably more physically friendly and have fewer limitations as well as less damaging effects than others – older people can still enjoy the benefits derived from swimming and cycling (non-weight bearing activities); however, few of the elderly enjoy the act of running! For me, because I train daily and race regularly, physiological sporting changes come very slowly – tomorrow is currently the same as yesterday, and as mentioned changes are only really apparent in race results. Leading up to and including the age of 61 years of age, my cycling performances were exemplary, but thereafter, and the closer I got to 70, the more obvious were the changes. Looking back, when I was 61 years of age I raced a 10-mile cycling time trial in 20m 25s (and was disappointed to find I hadn't gone under 20), now that's very close to 30mph cycling on public roads and facing the inclement northern weather; the same year I also rode a couple of 25 mile time trials in 54m 34s (same exact time twice, different courses) and was still bucking the trend as I continued to ride 'steel framed' heavier bikes, with few 'go quicker' fairings, and as always with the sport of cycling my recovery after 'flat-out' races was almost *instantaneous* (give me a slurp of tap water or milk, and I'll go again – please! sums it up). Thereafter, i.e. after 61 years of age, there has been a gradual but obvious (and somewhat baffling – to the sporting mind) drop in cycling performances most years, right up to the current year, 2021 where at 70 I had been initially struggling to go under 24 minutes for a 10-mile Time Trial (24m 10s, 24m 12s, and 24m 13s) since those earlier events though, and having made training adjustments, I have lowered my season's best time to a current *23m 18s* (a full minute on a bike is a big improvement); all the latter events by-the-way were on the same identical course, a course which has eight roundabouts to negotiate! As my physical performances ease, 'maybe' I am becoming slightly more intelligent (surely not!!) because for the first time in my sporting life I am a cautious pussy-cat and I consciously go slower on roundabouts now than I would have done previously – a collision with a car or the impacting tarmac on my skeletal frame at 70 years of age resulting in 'breakages' or worse, is simply not worth another 45 seconds off my time, whereas younger riders, or so it seems, have little regard for the potential danger posed by Kamikaze drivers, speeding traffic, gravel or rain on the uncertain terrain that are roundabouts! On reflection, some of this year's (2021) poorer results may be contributed to not giving all my training time solely to improving racing on my bike, because I have also been running and swimming several times a week as well as biking 'every day' with the aim being to compete in Duathlon (run/bike/run races) and Aqua/Bike (Swim and bike races), and of the two races I've done *I have finished in the top 5 'overall' in both despite being officially in the 70 year old category;* these results were pleasing and at least indicated I once again got my prep right in terms of getting to the start line healthy (although with niggling injuries) and having good form on the day of the 'multi-sport performances'!

At the time of writing this chapter, I have cycled in some form every day from 3rd August 2020 (as from the 2nd August 2020 I had a running related Achilles problem, which prevented me running and I'd previously had 77 consecutive days of running up to the 2nd August) right up to today 21st August 2021, so that's 381 consecutive days, and tomorrow I am optimistically racing another 10! What I've learned is that as far as the bike is concerned, 'consistency' alone doesn't make you a faster athlete – I knew that already, of course – it's simple, if you want to race fast – you have to regularly train fast and the faster you train, the more recovery you will require afterwards, and resting has always been a problem for me. The more work I do, the more I want to do, similar I suppose to other 'addicts' such as the alcoholic or the drug taker, both of whom seemingly also crave more; hard work is habit forming and although there are clearly positives there are also many negatives. With steady state consistent training you build stamina and enhance motor-skills but not necessarily increased speed, subjecting the racing body to racing conditions is a very important part of progression (training should be *progressive, consistent* and *specific* to the aim); however, on a more positive note, the more consistent your training is, the quicker you return to racing form perhaps after an injury, apathy or the winter's 'lull'!

As important, but rarely mentioned or considered, is the issue of *'physical athletically induced pain'* (see following chapter entitled Roll-up etc.) during competitions, and that is always the same – extreme pain due to extreme effort, which is driven I suppose more by athlete mentality than athletic ability – competitions hurt like hell, always did and still do, anyone who enters a competition and is not in 'some sort of effort based pain' is not racing. Having said the latter, the stopwatch never lies and cursing it gets us nowhere, absolutely no argument, 'truth' as confirmed by the cheap plastic time-piece on my sweaty wrist is a big leveller and replacing the old 'slow' watch with a 'more reliable' new 'faster' one is really clutching at straws – whispering, with a bit of positive 'self-talk' – such as, *'I'll go faster today – I have a new watch'* only makes sense after several pints of Guinness!

And so it seems you have several options as you age *if you are a racing competitor:* you can continue to race and become increasingly sad and frustrated at your perceived inadequacy to perform as you used to as other competitors who were once slower now pass with apparent ease before gradually disappearing over the horizon. Alternatively, you can try to at least maintain last year's results, or you can give-in and ease the pain somewhat by resting on your laurels whilst quietly murmuring *'I'm done,* I've been lucky, *you've had a good innings, Michael old son, be sensible, you're a grandad, move on'* before you finally sever your racing links all together and say **enough!** Then join an R&B band and keep fit by carting tube amplifiers around after midnight!

In biblical terms, *'three score years and ten'* has a certain ring to it, and whoever wrote that term knew what they were talking about, suggesting as it does that everything has a variable although quite predictable lifespan. Another factor, for me at least, is that with every year or two from around 63 years onwards there has been a decline in performance, which becomes more profound after 65; certainly at 70 I'm not the same athlete I was at 65, 66, 67, or even, so it seems at 68 and 69 – doesn't make sense, because in real terms it's only yesterday; regardless, times are an undeniable truth as well as an irrefutable statement of fact. When I was younger, my body and mind were one, a great match, my mind dictated and my body simply nodded its acceptance! I can see no difference, results-wise, between being 21 and 41; indeed my best athletic years were between 35 and 40, I was winning British Championships and continuing to get stronger and quicker. I left triathlon when I was 43 with a disappointing

8th place in Guernsey in the National long course Championships that year. Soon after my triathlon years I was competing in Ultra-fit competitions and then racing on the bike where I won loads of races during a 12 year spell right up to 60, regularly beating fit people half my age. And now? Well, in athletic terms I have been through the mill, a total understatement – has anyone done more or gone as quick? A huge statement – but I'm serious! A return to triathlon after a lengthy absence (and therefore the re-commencement of the impactive activity of 'running') when I was 63 was perhaps my biggest sporting challenge; however, a 'never say die' attitude had me running 57 x 5km Park Runs with an overall 'average' of 19m 47s as well as top 3 placings! My last ones were when I was touching 69! Maybe I just got lucky!

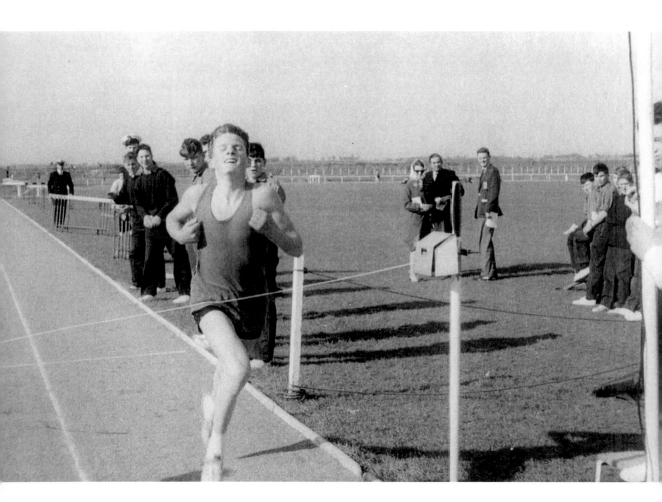

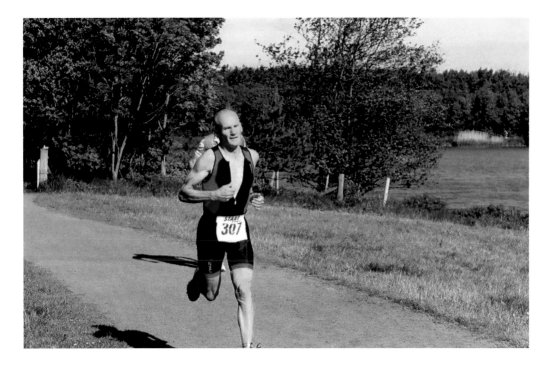

A mile in 04:48 as a 15 year old (1967), slightly slower as a 68 year old (2019) but the effort is identical.

Condensing the whole and it looks like this. At 15 years of age as a Junior Seaman, I ran 4m 48s for a mile on an accurate purpose-built 1950s style uneven 440yd cinder track in the trainers which I'd earned by plucking Christmas turkeys on Jacky Herdman's farm (remember that); I didn't have spikes. At the time at HMS Ganges I was running a maximum of three days of 'stolen' or 'unauthorised' running training a week, when my ship mates did 'make and mend' duties (uniform maintenance) I'd quietly slink out the Mess door and somehow incorporate 30 minute running training into the life of a very busy Junior Seaman in the Royal Navy. Now here we are 54 non-stop energetic and athletic years later and at 69 years of age as a 'not so busy' retired gent and I was running six-minute mile pace for 3,000metres but this time on an up-front, nothing to hide, seven days of authorised running training a week as opposed to the three days of stolen running back in 1967. That sort of example straight off the top of my head, just about sums up the *youth and age* physical performance debate – I mean you don't get 70-year-old athletes running 4m 48s mile races or winning Olympic gold medals UNLESS perhaps partnered by a super-fast pedigree of a horse with a shiny coat and bushy tail!

But on a real positive note, forget physical performance for a minute, athletic performance can be about so much more than fast times and winning performances, it's also about remaining healthy as well as being physically able, if, that is, you take a *holistic* path to health, combining both exercise with healthy nutrition; additionally, it's also a clear portrayal of a person's character, advertising to the world issues such as determination, effort, discipline and somewhere within all of those traits finding a degree of personal pride and contentment, all of which can add positively to our lives! *Once again those views are simply for consideration, as well as in line with this publication and the title which includes '70 years of experimentation'!*

So, before moving on, where am I now? Well I'm clearly no Billy Shakespeare; however, maybe I'm best summed up this way!

I am similar to an old relic of a VW Beetle, a car once renowned for its longevity, and I've had three of them, a car that has 250,000 miles on the clock of the 'original' factory-fitted engine!

Just like the old Beetle, and despite the countless miles it's covered, I can still cruise comfortably or aerobically at 60mph; alas, I'm no longer capable of accelerating anaerobically from 0 – 60 in 10 seconds, nor am I comfortable performing right on the aerobic/anaerobic threshold at 80mph as I once was, even with a tail wind! However, similar to the respected vehicle, I am, if nothing else, both reliable and infinitely dependable on the basis that if I turn up and I'm capable of moving, I'll always give my best. My mind-set and my abnormal healthy human cardio-vascular-system, just like the functioning VW engine, continues to propel my aging body very efficiently even as the body continues to slowly deteriorate whilst it enters into an unpredictable and unknown territory. Good job there are no human MOTs though, as one of those would invariably see us both, the Beetle and me, scrapped!

Back briefly to Mr Shakespeare's wondrous inspiring words which opened this chapter – and his take on mankind with – what a piece of work is a man, 'in form and moving how express and admirable, how like an angel, the beauty of the world, the paragon of animals!' **AT 20, well maybe, at 70 Ha! I think not, give me a pint of what he was drinking!! 'HE SHOULD HAVE GONE TO SPEC-SAVERS!' What say you my reliable learned friend –** Davy Gray?

STILL WITH ME? READ ON!

ROLL UP, ROLL UP, ROLL UP!

TAKE YOUR SEAT, LADIES AND GENTS FOR THE 'ATHLETIC' CLASH OF THE DECADE!

IN THE RED CORNER WE HAVE OUR CARDIO-VASCULAR SYSTEM – AND IN THE BLUE CORNER WE HAVE OUR SKELETAL AND MUSCULAR FRAME!

Current odds at Ladbrokes = 1-5 on in favour of?

For the past handful of years my head (the governor) has *refereed* a constant and on-going battle, a war if you like, between two quite different and severely contradictory foes, and the two enemies continually haggle and argue. The contest here is between my phenomenally efficient and athletically wonderful *Cardio-vascular System* in the 'red corner' and in the 'blue corner' there's my highly developed but aging or elderly *muscular system and skeletal frame*, from which it all hangs. Now as we all know, most battles arise from a 'difference of opinion' where two sides argue over perceived discrepancies, one saying one thing whilst the other side counters and disagrees while saying something totally different. Sometimes the more powerful of the two parties wins the contest; however, in contrast, sometimes the cleverer or more determined of the two takes the prize! For me, I try hard to listen and interpret both sides of my body but it's difficult because the 'red' corner is so very different from the equally persistent 'blue' corner! The 'red' corner urges me to *'keep going, you can do better, go quicker, travel for longer, you've done it all before, now come on you're loafing, you're barely out of breath, so pick it up, Tosser'!* The 'blue' corner keeps butting-in and continually interrupts shouting *'are you mad, slow down, you simpleton, remember you've never been that bright, it was your sister who went to Grammar School in a proper uniform, you were always a bit thick now, weren't you – be honest, why don't you listen to me, go slower, man, or you'll get yet another injury, you aren't capable – ouch, told you!'*

Currently my personal battle is between two sides of my body whose whole aim and directive in life was only ever designed and intended to work 'closely together' and in unison for the good of the whole. The problem is simple: my Cardio is just 'superb' – if I could sell it, I'd make a million overnight; in contrast, if selling my body (neck down) on eBay – I'd get nowt! Improving your cardio, you see, is really quite easy: all you need is movement; however, trying to make tired and elderly muscles and bones more efficient is a different kettle of fish. For example, today (and it's a normal Wednesday, on the 5th May 2021) I ran seven miles on Stobswood field; admittedly it was slow because I'm tentatively returning from a running-related injury so I'm only averaging 8m 30s miles, I am barely breathing, and I'm pleased in my solitude that no-one is watching – I mean, I was a decent runner once! After the running I returned home and immediately sat on my 'indoor' rust bucket of a second-hand 20 year old exercise bike for 45 minutes where I averaged between 92 and 98 rpms. For my cardio it was 'oh so very easy', I even read the newspaper at the same time as I pedalled and 'attempted' the frustrating crossword (I know all the answers but they frustrate me by hiding!). After the latter, I did my usual strength exercises, press-ups using bars, dips, curls, shoulder press, abs and core, followed by a well-rehearsed stretching routine. As mentioned, my breathing in the 'red' corner was *exemplary*, so much so I could have sat an 'easy' GCSE during the workout. I could have made love to five young maidens (or maybe even five older not so young women – PC savvy, eh?) while laughing hysterically at the joy of it all, and still not broke sweat; I could have had tea and ginger snaps with the Queen and then danced the 'dashing white sergeant' with her if she was in the mood!' Or even gyrated sexily to the Twist, that's Chubby Checkers' classic, if she'd had a Guinness and was in good fettle!

Oh, but the other side in the 'blue' corner doesn't play the game in the same way. In a nutshell, and in contrast to my cardio (in the red corner), my legs hurt! My left Achilles is worrying, I have a 'Glute' problem that comes and goes, and despite running on grass and on flat terrain my right shin is also concerning and if I'm not mistaken 'shin-splints' beckon? And all of that is so predictable and all down to 'running' on an elderly, much-used frame, because on the bike I can ride for two hours 'flat-out' (I've rode every single day since August last year and it's currently May 2021) and feel nothing except occasional 'exhilaration' deriving from the often 'intense – take-no-prisoners – effort', that's the reward that comes with a non-weight bearing activity. **<u>But</u>** I'm leaned on, because when I feel as if I'm running well it's a difficult to explain joy and I love the freedom of it, I always did, hence I keep returning, and regardless of the developing stiffness when I finish, I have a contented smile.

Talking 'pain'! This is what I've found:

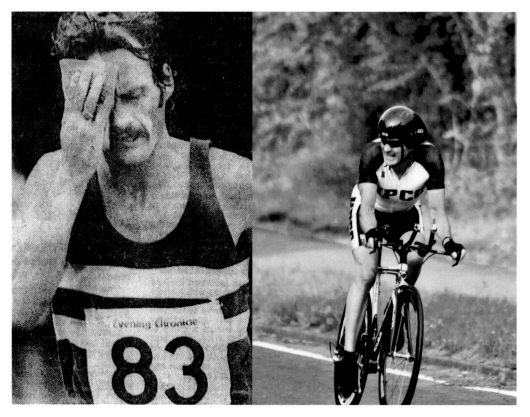

Whether winning marathons or time trials, the face says it all!

There are different 'severities' of athletically induced pain (forgive my terminology if it isn't textbook perfect) which are difficult to quantify. There are 'lesser' (discomfort) and 'greater' (intense physiological pain) degrees of pain influenced by both physical fitness levels and mental tolerance levels. BUT when you are 'flat-out' there is no guesswork involved based on the fact that however you are performing, you are incapable of giving more. However, 'regardless of age', when you are working 'flat-out' whether you are 16 or 70, the extremes of pain are 'identical' based on the premise that you are unable/incapable of giving more. The younger athlete wins the race, not because they can withstand more pain than the older athlete (both athletes are feeling the same grotty intensity), but the younger pulls away and wins by a margin simply because the energy, power output, and speed they can generate is far greater than the old fella simply due to their youth; *a new Formula 1 will always beat an old Ford Anglia even if Lewis Hamilton is behind the wheel of the Ford!* Some young athletes can run, cycle and swim at 90-95 percent of their maximum (and raise it again 'very' briefly for that final sprint to the tape) and their 'maximum' heart rate may be as high as 220bpm and for some trained individuals that could mean they are operating on 180 plus bpm. The older 'has-been athlete' can be flat out as well, giving the exact 'same effort' as their younger counterpart, yet their pulse rate hovers 'only' around 155bpm and for him/her that is also 95 percent of their max, so regardless, their output in terms of energy, power, speed is miles apart! *Another thing, particularly with early start competitions, is that the older athlete is 'slow' to warm-up, we don't particularly enjoy early starts, we are regularly stiff first thing and are easily 'thumped' by oxygen debt!*

The great thing with keeping training diaries, and I've 45 plus, is that you can return to them at will and compare today's efforts with last year's, or five years ago and 20 years ago and so on; the information is spellbinding! Recently I did a biking interval session 'indoors' so there was no weather issues, I was using the same antiquated rusty machine I've used for 20 years – you could catch more disease off this thing than a Bigg Market toilet, I kid you not. I did a 30-minute spin warm-up, then did 20x30 seconds flat-out efforts on a big gear (number 12) with 30 second spin recovery on gear 6 between all efforts. My revs per minute for the efforts were 104, and 90rpm for the recovery spin on gear 6. On conclusion I did a 10-minute cool-down to finish. At the end of the session I was 'in awe of myself' being able to work at that rate at 69 years of age – UNTIL later that night I looked at a training diary from 10 years previously (when I was 59 – but still 'winning' cycle races) and discovered I was then doing 20x1minute (not 30s ones) flat-out efforts at 1 minute intervals, but then working at 114 rpms on gear 12. In both instances the pain was identical because I was working flat-out – in both cases I couldn't have given more. It was the 10 year age gap which was the decider, and clearly there is nothing I can do about that except sigh, shake my head laterally and smile!

I mentioned Personal Bests times when talking about Park Runs in an earlier chapter and how special they are for each of us. Most athletes are the eternal optimists, no one more so than me, one of the reasons for my optimism was that because my cardio was so special, within seconds of finishing a race and despite the effort, I was able to hold a conversation, that always led me to believe there was more to come. I once lost my British title in a sprint finish by three seconds (over a two hour race), the other guy (the victor) was rolling all over the ground in apparent agony as the press flocked around him bulbs flashing endlessly, I walked away despondent but in full control. The question then was did I give enough? Or was I just a slower sprinter? I like to believe I was slower in the final 50 metres, if I'd had a coach he would have said you left it too late – learn by it, don't leave it till the end. Here's a thing, when I was at my best, most of my times were very similar. I once did two 10-mile time trials (bike), a week in between, and both times were identical 20m 41s, on public roads! Many years later I did three Park Runs when I was 68 at the same venue, on three consecutive Saturdays, 18m 57s, 19m 06, 19m 05s – being rational it would appear I was going probably as quick as I was capable. Most people don't shed minutes off their times when they get a new PB, they shed seconds!!

Back to the present. A little over a year ago I was running six-minute miles, 11 minutes on a measured road course with other much younger athletes, the distance was an accurate 3km and I was a hair's breadth from being 69 years of age that day; more to the point I was convinced I would soon go much quicker!! The challenge for me and no doubt many others is simply to continue to run and remain injury free, it's yet another 'call to fight', can it be done? Who will be the victor? – the simple answer I feel is yes, it is feasible, providing I'm prepared to slow my running down, run less, and run on the cushion that is grass for the most part. The alternative is to ride the bike and continue to surprise myself, not just with quality results but also with a vigour and longevity which defies my age. Another alternative is to take a more holistic view and 'Cross Train' (see earlier chapter), adding more variety, such as swim, bike, run, walk, etc, etc.

Still talking age, as far as *exercise* is concerned, the over 60s, or so I've discovered, are a forgotten category, which is one of the reasons for writing this late in the day book, and that's in contrast to the young, smiling, visually pleasing media models who demonstrate with such vigour all the expensive fitness apparatus all of which is aimed at the same youthful age category as themselves. When was the last time you saw similar fitness products advertised by a 60-something 'model'? It is exceedingly 'rare' (an understatement) to see a television advert aimed solely at the 60-plus age group with fitness equipment. In fact, the only adverts aimed directly at the over 60s are for people with bad legs (legs that to all intents are 'broken' because, similar to old wheels – they don't work properly). Add to the latter those over 60 who have circulatory problems, perhaps hindered further by bad backs and dodgy knees, and those who can no longer chew claggy toffee because their dentures are no longer stuck down firmly enough, and worse those whose dentures are no longer cosmetically brilliant white, nor do their gobs smell like the freshness of Toilet Duck, Domestos or Polo Mints. Then there's those with arthritis as well as others troubled by penile erection issues (whatever that is?) and others by all accounts who have 'dryness' eh! What about those who are encouraged to get a hearing aid and 'quick' because if you stall any longer you'll get Alzheimer's, and why not kill two birds with one stone and on your way home take out a life insurance policy. There are special 'reading lights' available with specially designed arm chairs – to fall asleep in, much more comfortable and reassuring if you've got your incontinent panties on! The latter is all tongue in cheek, of course, so *here's a more positive take on it all.*

As far as 'athletic' issues are concerned, the process of aging (and it's the one thing we've all got in common) need not be negative, nor need it be accompanied by pessimism. In today's society we see both men and women in their 60s and beyond running marathons, but we also see kids in their teens incapable of shuffling a quarter of the distance. Youth and age are merely words; it's the interpretation which is the issue. I believe maturity and youth are a state of mind. We are what we think we are, old or young, you determine your state (how many times have I said that?); certainly, I know young people who by action and thought are old, and old people who likewise are youthful despite their years.

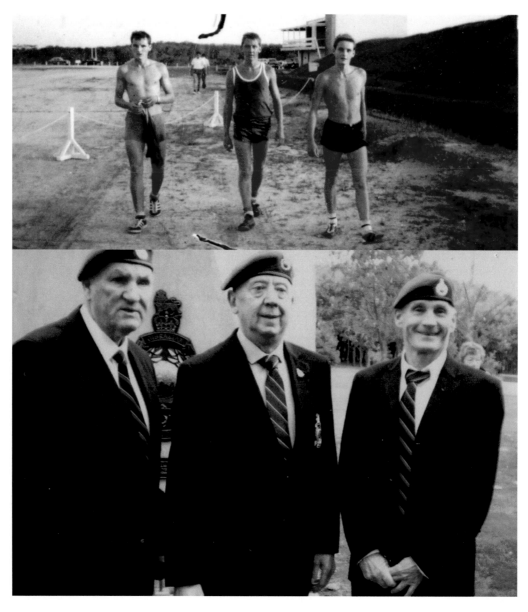

My good friends, Tommy Gunning, John Madden, and me following a 50 year gap

I'm guessing but maybe at least a half of our lives we benefit from our youth, we are in fact a 'new product'. As babies and through childhood we have a brand-new body which works in an exemplary fashion with few self-imposed physical limitations. On conclusion of youth (think of a figure!), and from that point onwards, we naturally begin to age but very slowly, although some age more rapidly than others. For many, as we age our once 'everything is possible' philosophy declines, for others the decline is an un-noticeable minimum. In our fourth decade and for those who value their vitality and continue to routinely service their health, they do age slower, some even become healthier and physically fitter as well as faster than they've ever been. In our 50s (remember I won 75-80 bike races all from the age of 50 up to and including 60 and even at 61 I rode 10 miles on an antiquated steel framed bike in 20m 25s – now that's 30mph!), there is no sudden catastrophic decaying process because of another birthday, and for some even in our 60s we are still very active whilst also cleaning with vigour our very own natural teeth. In contrast, some other people go on a television programme called *'a place in the sun'* and with pockets apparently full of money seek out their ideal retirement or holiday home. Then reality clicks in, they all want a swimming pool to go with the property, but only to sit beside and look at, most definitely don't want to swim in. They also want shops, but they've got to be 'really' close by, and without a hill, because they most definitely don't want to walk, and even if they did want to walk – they couldn't manage the hill or 'slight incline' anyhow, and so it goes on; I truly don't understand. Why go all the way to the tropics without a second language, to read a novel by the pool with a glass of warm coke, when you can do the very same at Whitley Bay with a cold coke, and there are buses there to take you to the town centre, and there's even the liberating North Sea – to look at of course!

Be an optimist, and have a good positive philosophy and state with a degree of sincerity and commitment *"next year I'm going to be much healthier and fitter than this year, that's for sure, and the year after I'll be even better!"* Is that possible? Of course it is, why not? Can I gain from that? Of course! Is it possible to get fitter and healthier as you get older? **Absolutely!!**

Acceptance, regarding health is static, it creates apathy, and apathy leads nowhere except perhaps to boredom, and boredom befriends no one. Acceptance is for the dead, those in graveyards. Us living people, well, we can 'still' choose, and the choice? We can physically deteriorate, we can remain where we are (temporarily), or we can progress and improve – come on, there's no contest, is there! The healthier and fitter we are the greater the possibilities and potential, and the fewer the limitations, age need not play such a significant or major role.

So be careful with tongue in cheek banter such as "I'm too old for all of this" because sooner or later you might just begin to believe it! And where does that negative banter leave you? Bloody well old!!! That's where.

Age isn't a disease, nor should it be feared, but to court it invites limitations, and limited beliefs create limited people, and limited people may ultimately be found wanting when opportunities beckon and choice is a necessity rather than a preference.

As mentioned somewhere above. Yesterday, I finished 5th in a Duathlon – I'm 70 and I truly believe that there's not another body on the planet that has been where mine has been in terms of athleticism!! But tomorrow and future years is unknown, which is probably just as well!! I might have to join a band, yep that sounds exciting!

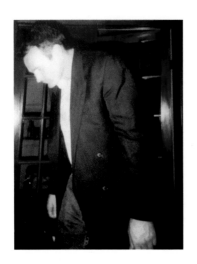

So after all of that, is there a definitive answer to staying physically fit and healthy? – Well it could be as simple as eating healthily and exercising with a smile and a laugh, regularly! GOOD LUCK!

After all of that, mine's a Guiness or three!!!

I started this book (inside of the front cover) with a frustrated almost political statement. As I write, Prince Philip has sadly just died. He apparently said, that being stationed in Malta in the late 1940s and early 1950s with his new bride the Queen was one of their happiest periods of the 75 years together. With my dad in the Royal Navy and posted in Malta during the same period, I just so happened to be born there in 1951. Being newly born, my parents and Linda my sister had the same draft as Prince Philip and his queen. Just along the coast from the Duke, I was a newly born little Geordie laddie just 'shitting' in the sun without a care in the world and about to begin such an athletic life; 70 years later I'm the same athlete although noticeably older – of course, but now 'domicile' in Widdrington.

Today Prince Philip was described amongst all the accolades as "not being very politically correct!" Well, his freedom of speech, comes with age, as does mine, I only hope mine is accepted with the same smiles and laughter as his royal highness's!!

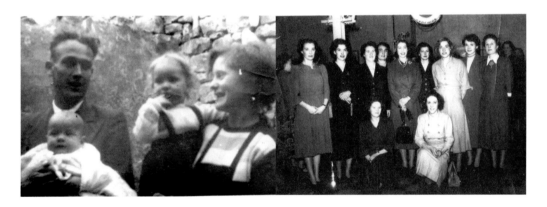

*This is us in Malta in 1951 and my mother
(kneeling, left) in front of the queen, same period.*

In October 2021 and on conclusion of 70 years of extreme physical living, the author has trained for 552 consecutive days. He has finished fifth overall in a duathlon (run/bike/run), fifth in an aqua/bike race (1500m swim/46km bike), rode 10 miles in a cycling time trial in 23m 18s, and after a two-year absence due to Covid and an Achilles injury, has finished in the top ten in his three Park Runs to date.

On reflection there are three things important in life, in any order you like: family, health, and friends – deduce from that what you will.

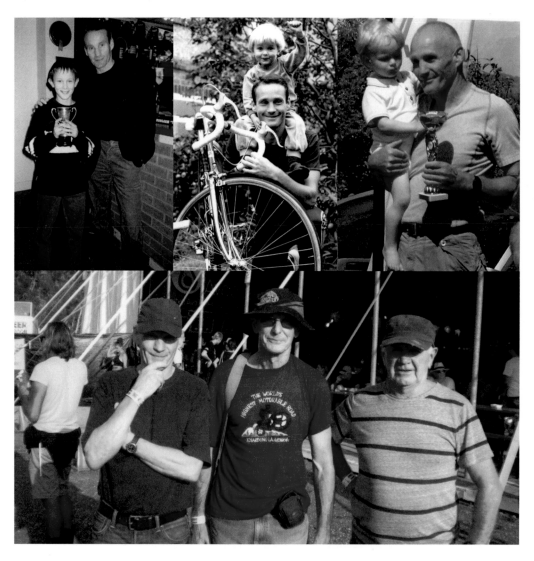

From five years to 70 years and from Stobswood to the Gold Coast, my good friends Jimmy and Ossie.

To **UK Book Publishing**, that's *Ruth, Jay, Judith* and *Dan*, my grateful thanks. I came back to you three times – which is a small but clear compliment! The 'returning' bit says it all.